LIFE IS TOUGH

BUT SO ARE YOU

HOW TO RISE TO THE CHALLENGE
WHEN THINGS GO PEAR-SHAPED

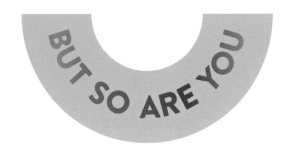

LIFE IS TOUGH

BUT SO ARE YOU

BRIONY BENJAMIN

murdoch books
Sydney | London

To you, dear reader

May this book be a
friend and a comfort
when life gets tricky.

Hello, dear reader

If you're reading this because your life has taken a tricky turn, I'm so sorry.

I wish I could reach through the pages of this book and give you a giant hug and we could sit down to have a cup of tea and talk it all through. This setback hasn't 'happened for a reason' or been sent to you because 'you're one of the strong ones', (cue eye roll). It's just crappy bad luck and it's totally not fair that you have to go through this.

This 'crappy bad luck' might take the form of a health crisis, a gut-wrenching loss, overwhelm and burnout, a mental health struggle, a broken heart, cancer or your own personal smorgasbord of unexpected life events.

And while you wouldn't have picked this out of the catalogue of life (duh), know that you can get through these tough times and emerge richer and stronger than before.

If you're reading this to support someone else (hello, friend of the year!) these pages will give you heaps of ways to help those you love navigate the tricky seasons. And it will give you some tips and tricks to keep up your sleeve for when life throws you an unexpected sucker punch.

When I was diagnosed with cancer at age 31, it was the shock of my life. I thought cancer only happened to people in the movies; like Mandy Moore in *A Walk to Remember*, or the hot Irish guy from *P.S. I Love You*. Suddenly I was the lead character in a film I didn't want to be in, without the cheesy love story.

After the initial shock wore off, I decided that if I had to do this I may as well make it as enjoyable as possible. Of course it wasn't all high fives and jazz kicks, but I was fortunate to get through it and I like the person it's made me become. I feel grateful for the early wake-up call that this is my one precious life. Sure, next time I want to reflect, I'll opt for the yoga retreat in Bali, but a major crisis is one hell of a way to make you focus on what really matters.

This book compiles all the most helpful and practical gems I learned along the way that made the whole experience more doable and less crap. Whatever it is that you or a loved one are going through, this book is here to provide comfort and strength and cheer you on from the sidelines. And to remind you that you've got this. Because, yes, life might be tough, but guess what? So are you!

love Briony B xx

Some crap things you might be experiencing right now

(SHITTIEST LIST IN THE HISTORY OF THE WORLD)

OVERWHELM
& BURNOUT

DIVORCE

DEPRESSION

ANXIETY

FERTILITY
ISSUES

BROKEN
HEART

CHRONIC
FATIGUE

CANCER

FINANCIAL HARDSHIP

MISCARRIAGE

JOB
LOSS

GRIEF

HEALTH
CRISIS

Contents

How to use this book

Well, it's your book: you do whatever you damn well want with it! Take it to the beach, lend it to a friend, leave it on your bedside table, spill coffee on it, mark pages that are helpful. You can read it in one go or dip in and out of it when you need a hit of inspiration, strength or some comfort and guidance.

When you see text in this box, it is a question for you to ponder or an activity to do.

If you're feeling overwhelmed, you don't have to manage on your own. There's a full list of helpful phone numbers and resources at the back of the book, starting on page 195.

An asterisk like this means there are links to evidence-based research, which you'll find in the back of the book (see pages 198–199).

PS. If you want to scribble along, I've made you a little gift in the form of a free workbook
download it at brionybenjamin.com.au

Introduction

Where it all began

The day before my life flipped upside down, I was at work in the Mamamia office – that's the digital platform for women, not *Mamma Mia!*, the musical. I was Executive Producer of Video and I loved my job: it was seriously fun, getting to come up with amusing and impactful video ideas, star in them and often watch them go viral. I'd meet and interview celebrities and experts as well as work on high-level digital strategy; not to mention the never-ending supply of cakes, treats and freebies that rolled in the door from brands and clients (it was very hard to be #sugarfree in that office).

I worked with a team of the most gorgeous and kind women I'd ever come across, who were whip-smart, hilarious and always stylishly dressed – normally in some combination of designer clothing and sneakers, and often featuring lots of sequins and sparkle. On this day in particular I'd curled my long blonde hair. I'd just had a spray tan and was wearing bright colours and bright lippy to compensate for feeling like a heavily caffeinated zombie. I remember my effervescent boss Mia Freedman walking past my desk in a characteristic fully sequined number and saying, 'Gosh, you look amazing!'

'Thanks. It must just be the spray tan,' I joked.

I might have looked good, but on the inside, I felt rotten.

Feeling awful had become my new normal. I was so used to always being a bit icky and tired that I had started to believe that this is how I would always feel. Perhaps this is what becoming an adult felt like? I had become an expert at compartmentalising pain, putting on a smile and just carrying on. When people would ask me how I was, I'd reply 'I'm great!' because it had become really boring, month after month, saying to friends and colleagues 'Ugh! I feel awful/sick/tired/like an achy deflated balloon.' Or if I did say that, they'd often reply, 'Yeah, I feel really tired too,' and so I just stopped telling them. I didn't want to be Briony the Buzzkill.

Besides, the doctors were telling me I was fine, that perhaps I was just 'stressed' and needed to rest more. But no matter how much I rested, meditated, ate vegetables, Marie Kondoed my room, drank the recommended water intake, stopped trying to consume the entire internet before bed, cut alcohol/caffeine/sugar/dairy/gluten/anything remotely fun, took vitamins and did mindfulness puzzles, I could just never get on top of the pervasive tiredness that had become a constant in my life. I was having sweats at night and always felt a bit crappy, but otherwise I appeared quite healthy. My body was sending me all the signs, but I didn't yet know how to listen and trust it.

Oh hello
curveball,
I did not see
you coming!

A BRIEF HISTORY OF FEELING CRAPPY

I FEEL AWFUL

NAH, YOU'RE JUST STRESSED

learn to MEDITATE

HMMM ...
NOW I HAVE
NIGHT SWEATS

COULD BE
HORMONES

HMMM ...
IT'S NOT MENOPAUSE;
YOU'RE ONLY 31

MAYBE I SHOULD DO A
JUICE CLEANSE?

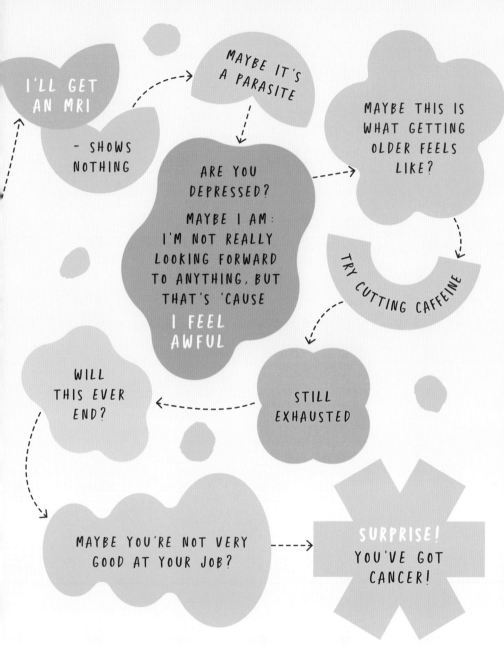

A very busy and important day

THURSDAY (very busy) to-do list

> Medical appointment 9am

> Uber to office

> Facebook Live with Bachelorette Sophie Monk

> Check set-up: audio & 2 cameras

> Complete video presentation

> Groceries on way home

I found myself sitting in the waiting room at the Prince of Wales Hospital in Sydney one very normal Thursday morning to get yet another set of test results. After a year of feeling really crappy, my parents insisted I go to a haematologist (a blood specialist) to get another opinion. I thought it was overkill, but I agreed. The specialist ordered some scans, more blood tests and a biopsy, and I didn't really think too much about it. Surely if the news was bad, they'd call straight away?

A week later I was there to get the results, expecting another dead end. Mum had insisted on flying down from Queensland and coming to the appointment with me, despite my protests. I was just going to race straight to work afterwards, I was too busy to hang out and had a jam-packed day. I figured it was a waste of a trip for her.

As I sat there with Mum waiting for my number to be called, I scrolled through work emails and planned the day ahead. I wondered how bad the traffic would be and how late I'd get into the office. My ticket number flicked up on the screen, so I put my phone away and Mum and I made our way down the corridor where we met Dr Annmarie Bosco. She greeted us warmly at the door of her brightly lit, white-walled office and welcomed us to take a seat.

Gently she said, 'So we need to discuss the results of the biopsy, it does show the Hodgkin's lymphoma your parents were concerned about. I'm so sorry.'

I took a sharp breath in, not yet comprehending what this meant. She explained that it was a type of cancer of the lymph glands, part of the body's immune system.

Cancer? What?

She gave me a moment to process the shock. Mum reached for my hand and held it tightly as we looked at each other in disbelief.

'You'll need to start treatment as soon as possible, so we will need you to clear your next three to six months. And, yes, it can be cured.'

To gauge how bad it was, I could only think of one question: 'Will I lose my hair?'

'Yes,' she said kindly, 'but it will grow back.'

My initial thoughts went something like this:

WTF?????????

Clearly there has been a mistake!

How can this be happening?

My hair...

But I'm so young?

There has definitely been a stuff-up.

OMG I'm going to be bald...

This is a pretty good excuse for being late to work.

How am I going to tell my sisters?

Perhaps they switched my results with someone else.

How am I going to tell my boyfriend?

No wonder my squash game has gotten so bad.

What if I have a weird-shaped head?

My hair, my beautiful hair: this can't be real.

How am I going to tell my friends?

Is this a prank?

Can I start today over?

FAAAAA

The rest of that consultation is a blur. I was so grateful that Mum had ignored me and come to the appointment (let's call it mother's intuition). She held my hand tight, we called Dad and put him on speakerphone and Dr Bosco gently talked us through the immediate next steps. More tests. Blah blah blah … IVF … Blah blah blah … I took out a pen and pad to take notes, but my mind was already somewhere else. Everything slowed down and a calm numbness came over me.

As I left the consultation, I looked down at my notepad. The only thing I'd written down was, 'don't get pregnant'. Helpful.

Nothing else that had seemed important that day mattered anymore. I held Mum's hand as we walked out of the hospital into the warm sunshiny Sydney day, where surprisingly the world hadn't stopped. Frantic people rushed by, disposable coffee cups in hand, glued to their phones; cars honked, their stressed drivers racing around doing their busy and important things. Didn't they know none of it mattered?

In a daze, Mum and I walked to a pharmacy on a bizarre expedition to buy pregnancy vitamins (more on this later).

I took out my phone, but this time it was to call all the people who were most important to me, one by one. Stuff racing off to work, we decided instead to go and have lunch by the sea, sit in the sunshine and watch the waves roll in. None of these things had been on my to-do list that morning. Hello curveball.

RRRRRRKKKKKKKKKKKKKKKKKKKKKKKKKK!!!!!!

Sometimes the universe will throw you a giant surprise party ... and, like most surprise parties, it's generally f%^king awful.

Things that mattered instantly

- Connecting with my favourite people on Earth
- How many days I had left on this planet
- Doing something important with that time

Things that instantly didn't matter anymore

- The 782 unread emails in my inbox

- My asymmetrical eyebrows (ladies' eyebrows are sisters, not twins)

- Being late to work

- My freckled white skin

- A presentation I had to give for work next week

- The aggro guy who road-raged at me this morning

- Getting fired from that job I didn't even really like ...

- What car I drove

- Missing out on the Year 12 drama award (nah, who am I kidding? That still cuts deep)

- My outfit for next week's party, to which I wouldn't be going anyway ...

- Who won *The Bachelorette*

THIS WASN'T ON MY VISION BOARD

The beginning of any crisis can be a bit of a blur.
Here are a few things that helped me in the early
days after my cancer diagnosis.

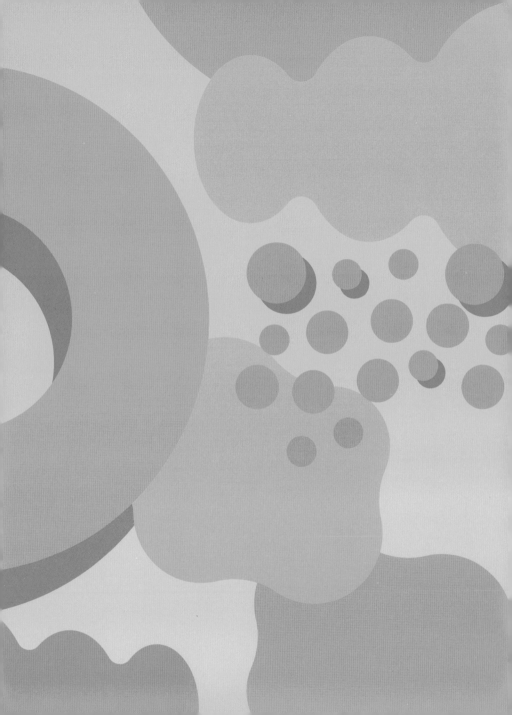

Day by day, step by step, breath by breath

The one piece of advice I do remember clearly from my specialist after she'd delivered the news that I had cancer was not to get too far ahead of myself. Dr Bosco suggested that I shouldn't google Hodgkin's lymphoma or worry too much about treatment just yet. Instead, we were just going to focus on the next few things we had to do. That was really excellent advice.

She gave me a piece of paper with the next steps written on it.

> blood tests

> heart & lung capacity tests

> appointment at the IVF clinic

In those first few days, as the enormity of what lay in front of me hit me in waves, I kept coming back to that. What are the next three steps?

It's a great way to approach anything in life. You don't have to solve everything right now, particularly when you are in crisis; you don't need to know where this will all lead. Things will unfold.

I use this all the time now, if I feel overwhelmed or stressed or anxious. What are the next few steps? Just focus on those.

I'm just going to take this one little step at a time

While we want to dream big and think big and know where we're going, sometimes we just need to break it down, focus on the next few things and take it day by day.

NINJA TIP

Remember, when it all gets too much, just take it day by day, step by step, breath by breath. (Oh, and try not to google too much.)

Get your pen and paper out, write down a list of the next things you need to do, and circle the three most urgent or important. Just focus on those. Everything else is going to wait its turn.

Some things don't have to be understood, just accepted

When you get bad news it's easy to want to know every single thing that has led to this. Whose fault is it? When did this begin? How long has this been going on? Why has this happened to me? I mean, c'mon, I'm a good person ... I eat healthily, I don't smoke, I always remember my re-usable bags, I've never ghosted on a date, I even do volunteer work, why me?

But that is EX-hausting. It's a great way to zap your energy and it doesn't help you to face the task ahead. Acceptance, hard as it can be, is key.

My wise friend Marieke, who had been through a huge life crisis herself, told me in those first few days, 'Remember, some things don't have to be understood, just accepted.' She sent me a slightly altered version of the well-known Serenity Prayer and suggested that I light a candle, sit in the dark and find a way to accept what was happening.

Serenity Prayer
Grant me the serenity
to accept the things
I cannot change
Courage to change
the things I can
And the wisdom to
know the difference.

These words helped me a lot in my first week after diagnosis. It's so true: some things are just random crappy bad luck. They don't happen for a reason, they're not part of some greater plan, it's just chaos theory. That's life. Try not to waste any energy on 'why me?' There is no answer. All you can do is accept it and then make a plan to move forward.

A shining example of this was the story of a dear family friend, Jeff Thorpe, who was diagnosed with Motor Neurone Disease (MND) around the same time I got my diagnosis. MND is a terrible disease that slowly degenerates the nerve cells that control the muscles that allow you to move, speak, breathe and swallow. The average life expectancy from diagnosis is a couple of years. Despite the initial shock and sadness, Jeff never once asked, 'Why me?' Instead he always said, 'Why not me?' He faced his final years with such grace and strength and was the most brilliant example to me of not wasting any time feeling sorry for yourself. I will forever remember his sunny and kind disposition until the very end.

As hard as it is, once you're ready you can try to accept the things that are beyond your control. Surrender to the circumstances, because in a way a crisis is a bit like a mammoth swim: you have to keep swimming, or at least go with the current, even when you don't feel like it.

Light a candle, sit in the stillness and surrender. Can you find a way to accept this shitstorm?

Braver, stronger, smarter

It's easy to be brave when life is smooth sailing, when you've had everything go your way, but when the storm comes, that's when you really get to see what you are made of. The good news is that resilience isn't something you are given at birth (or not): you can build your resilience. You will rise to the challenge because you have to. It's what we humans do and have done for as long as life has existed. And it can be interesting to see what you are made of.

There are oceans inside you. A vastness, a depth, a grit that you may not yet know exists within. You will have moments and days that will throw you off kilter and you won't be sure if you've got what it takes, but I promise you can learn.

Take a moment to remember that you are not alone. Many people before you have overcome extraordinary adversity. You are strong, you can and will overcome this (even if it sometimes sucks balls).

Take the words of the Serenity Prayer on page 16 and write an action plan; for example, 'Grant me the serenity to accept that I've lost my job; the courage to get out there and market myself; and the wisdom to know that I'm not a failure. (I'm freakin' awesome.)'

You've got this.

You'll basically be Tony Robbins by the end of this

Yep, tough times are totally awful. For sure! One major flipside is that you will morph into a giant motivational guru by the end. Seriously, the world is full of self-professed life coaches; however, you – my friend – are going to come out of this as the real deal.

I spoke to my friend Luke before I started treatment, because he was the only person I knew who was my age and had gone through chemotherapy. He'd had testicular cancer a few years earlier. He told me I would emerge from this experience stronger, richer and wiser than ever with a really clear understanding of life and what matters. (If someone else had said that to me, my eyes probably would have rolled out of my head.) But Luke had the cred – and the stitches – that allowed him to say that. In that conversation he handed me a cape and turned my sickness into a superpower.

Now I'm not saying I was excited to start chemotherapy after that little chat, but I certainly felt calmer approaching it with openness and a new-found curiosity. It somehow took away my fear and instead made me think, 'I'm going to be superhuman after this.' It flipped the crisis into an opportunity for growth.

In fact, psychologists Richard Tedeschi and Lawrence Calhoun coined the term 'posttraumatic growth' to articulate the positive psychological transformation that people can experience following a trauma or challenge: not only do people survive but oftentimes they thrive and grow from their experience. This is because an event that blows things up makes us reconsider everything, and that is necessary for human development and growth.

The great thing about going through shitty times is that it does embolden you. It makes you feel quite superhuman when you've gotten yourself through something enormous. I feel so much more free and strong these days: whenever I'm feeling a little shy or 'less than', if I am meeting someone or doing a presentation or in a crowd of particularly cool and intimidating people, I think, 'You guys have no idea what I've been through. I got through cancer, so this is a walk in the park.' I put my shoulders back, stand tall and think, 'This is not as scary as day one of chemo, so get over it and get on with it and don't let anyone dull your shine.'

NINJA TIP

The GREAT news is you don't have to wait for tragedy to strike to learn these lessons; you can build your resilience before a crisis comes along. I believe that building your physical and mental resilience while the sun shines is one of the greatest things you can do for yourself. For tips on how to do this, see pages 156–159 and 169–171.

You're going to be even more awesome on the other side, okay? Ain't nothing going to mess with you after this.

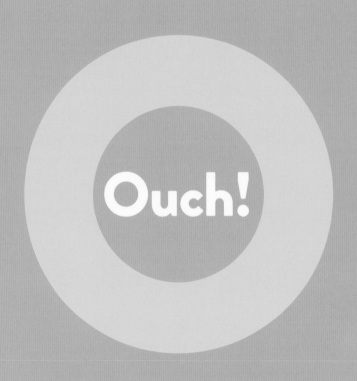

Universe,
I really did
not see that
coming ...
Where the hell
do I begin?

You don't have to be Pollyanna

Remember Pollyanna, the perky, optimistic little girl who found the good in absolutely everything? Like Pollyanna, when I was growing up I always prided myself on being optimistic and bubbly, no matter what. For now, though, screw Pollyanna. I'm letting you off the hook right here and right now. You are allowed to feel sad and scared and flat and angry when shit happens.

Remove the pressure straight away: you don't have to be positive and look for the silver lining in every moment. When I first found out I had lymphoma I remember thinking, 'Okay, I'm going to make this so much fun and I'm going to be so positive, I'LL BE THE MOST POSITIVE CANCER PATIENT ON THE PLANET!'

Losing my hair ... *it will grow back and maybe teach me to be less vain.*

Having to stop my work and my career ... *it will be nice to have a break.*

Packing up my flat and moving home ... *it will be nice to spend more time with Mum and Dad.*

Nice to have a break? Sweetie, this ain't a beach retreat, it's freaking chemotherapy and it freaking sucks. All of these things were really tough. Sure, there were heaps of people in WAY worse positions than me. But that didn't make my feelings any less valid. (It's not a crappiness competition.)

Feel the grief

I'm the first to acknowledge that good can come out of bad BUT you do not have to pretend to like this. You've GOT to feel what you feel! That's why they are called feelings.

In fact, it's good for us to sit in sadness and feel the grief. You're allowed to feel overwhelmed and sorry for yourself (for a little bit). If you do keep suppressing all of your emotions they will come back to bite you at some stage. There is nothing more annoying than someone telling you to 'just be positive': you literally want to punch them. And the same is true when speaking to yourself (but punching yourself is hard).

I saw a psychologist the week I was diagnosed and she said that I didn't have to enjoy any part of this experience or look for any positives, I could hate the whole thing if I wanted (geez, that was a bit extreme, I thought). But it released a pressure valve, knowing I was allowed to be sad. She gave me permission to sit on the couch and cry all day if I liked, but the next day I had to get up.

There is a fine line between feeling sad and wallowing in sadness that can be tricky to navigate. You're allowed to sit with it and let yourself feel what you need to feel, but don't be consumed by it. If you feel like you really can't get off that couch or might never want to ever again, then some professional help might be a good idea. In fact, I think it's a MUST when you've been thrown a curveball! (But more on that later.)

 Remember, it's okay to be scared and sad because it is scary and it is sad. Sit with it, have a cry, mourn the loss and know that your feelings are valid.

Welcome the pain in for a cup of tea

By this point you might think I've officially lost the plot. Welcoming pain? Are you mad? But hear me out. It's normal to want to push the pain away, sit on it, suppress it, strangle it or even ignore its very existence (just like how I feel about completing my tax return each year), but another approach is to lean into it. Welcome it in and make space for it rather than trying to fight it. Once you've accepted the pain and allowed yourself to feel sad, it's helpful if you can now make space for it.

Be it physical pain or emotional grief, try to make friends with it.

Welcome in the loneliness, the heartache, the grief, the pain – make space for it and just sit with it. Hell, give it a name if you want to. Maybe your loneliness is a Fred or that sick grief-stricken sadness you're feeling is more of a Horace. Well, Horace is a dick, but he's here whether you ignore him or not. Try thinking, 'Hello Horace, you're back again. No problems, come and have a seat.'

That might seem like very odd advice. It's like making friends with your least favourite person on the planet, and I'm not saying it's easy to do straight away. The idea is that instead of burning up precious energy hating and fixating on this foreign invader, there's now a lack of resistance there because you've made space for it, you are accepting it. It now can't exhaust you in the way it did before.

> What pain are you feeling at the moment? Are you pushing it away or ignoring it? Is there a way you can accept and acknowledge the pain and even try to make friends with the little jerk?

Approach it with a dash of 'she'll be right'

You've accepted what is happening. You've allowed yourself to feel what you're feeling and you've even made space for the pain. I found it helpful to have an overarching mentality of 'oh well, she'll be right'. Of course I wanted to survive (obviously), and live my life (I've got a lot of unfinished business to attend to), but I also needed to find a balance so I could conserve my energy, live lightly and not let it totally consume me.

Many of my good friends are campaigners and changemakers who care fiercely about creating a better, more equal society. The challenges they work with are mammoth, but if they focused only on the size of the problems they are up against, they'd feel so hopeless they wouldn't do anything. Instead, they understand the enormity of the problems and simply get on with the things they can do.

I think it's similar with a major life blow-up. You have to balance a deep passion and commitment for what you can do with a bit of detachment from the outcome.

Here are some other phrases that might work for you, or you might hate them! It's like a pick and mix: take what you like and leave the weird gross treats for someone else.

- Even the worst moments and feelings will pass.
- It is what it is.
- This is just a thing I'm going through right now.

Worry is like a rocking chair ...

... it gives you something to do, but gets you nowhere. I've tried to live by the philosophy of a dear family friend, Gary Wield. He believed that if you worry about something that doesn't eventuate, then you worried for no reason. But if you worry about something that does eventuate, then you have done double the worrying. So really the only way you can win is to wait until you are certain there is something to worry about. Then you can deal with whatever that is.

I figured throughout my experience that it was best not to worry, where possible, and instead just take it as it comes. Waaayyy easier said than done. But really worth a try, because needlessly worrying just drains you and depletes your energy.

> I'M NOT GOING TO WORRY ABOUT
  THAT ANY MORE TODAY.

> I'LL WORRY ABOUT THAT WHEN
  THERE IS A REASON TO WORRY
  ABOUT IT.

> IS THIS WITHIN MY CONTROL?
  IF NOT, THEN I WON'T WORRY
  ABOUT IT AT THIS POINT.

After chemo finished, I used to worry about the cancer coming back – it's a really common fear in cancer survivors. My beautiful friend Emily Somers, whom I met in the Land of Lymphoma, used to say to me: 'You know what? Your cancer could come back or it might not and whether or not you worry about it has nothing to do with it.' It helped, when I had appointments and check-ups, just to wait until I had concrete proof there was a problem before I started worrying about what to do.

As hard as it is, keep telling yourself, 'Future me is going to worry about that another day when I am certain there is something to worry about. And I will handle whatever is thrown my way.'

 Schedule in your worrying: 'Okay, I'm going to worry about that between 5.00 pm and 5.05 pm today; until then I will not think about it.'

PLOT TWIST: NOW WHAT?

Well, it's showtime. You're going to learn to ask
for what you need, and surround yourself with
a kick-arse team of humans so you feel supported,
strong and secure as you step into the next stage.

Your permission slip

If there has ever been a time you were allowed to ask for whatever you want, this is it! It's your crisis and there have to be a few perks, right? So revel in the golden, guilt-free permission slip to ask for what you want and need. (Space, quiet, snacks, a pet unicorn ...) Asking for what you need is something that is always available to us, but we don't often feel we can tap into it. Only you know what you truly need, and being able to articulate that to others is key.

In case, like me, you struggle with asking for what you need, here is a handy all-purpose everlasting permission slip to remind you of what you're allowed to ask for!

PERMISSION SLIP*

FROM THIS DAY FORWARD I HAVE FULL PERMISSION
TO DO WHATEVER FEELS RIGHT AND GOOD FOR ME;
TO ASK FOR WHAT I NEED; TO CREATE BOUNDARIES
ABOUT WHERE AND HOW I SPEND MY TIME AND ENERGY.

NUMBER OF REPEATS:
INFINITE. USE LIBERALLY WHENEVER YOU NEED IT.

EXPIRY DATE:
NEVER! THIS LASTS FOR A LIFETIME.

---

*Snap a photo of this permission slip and keep it on your phone to remind yourself that you are allowed to do what you please.

It might feel awkward to ask for what you want. Here are some suggestions of how to approach your friends and family, and some of the things you might find it helpful to ask for.

'Hey, lovely friend, thanks for reaching out and offering your support. To be honest I feel a little awkward asking, but here are some ideas of the things you could do for me right now.'

☐ Could you help coordinate everyone so that someone checks on me each day? I really need the support right now.

☐ Could you pick the kids up from school on Thursdays?

☐ Could you send me a text to check in on me every few days?

☐ Could you walk with me one morning each week?

☐ Could you please check in on the people who are looking after me?

☐ Could you drop off a meal one day a week? That would be such a help.

☐ Could you drop in and keep me company for a while?

☐ Could I have some quiet time, please?

☐ Can you water the plants?

☐ Can you take me to the moon? I really need to get outta here.

Highlight your current needs in the list above and send a snap of this page to a friend.

TAKE WHAT YOU NEED

SOME QUIET TIME

A DELICIOUS NAP

CUP OF TEA

SOMEONE TO CHECK IN WITH ME EACH DAY

PLAYFULNESS

A SUNNY SPOT TO SIT

A DOCTOR I TRUST

SOMEONE TO HOLD MY HAND

STABILITY

CHILLED PEOPLE AROUND ME

COMPASSION

A LITTLE CRY

PHYSICAL TOUCH

TO BE TOLD I AM LOVED

SOME GENTLE EXERCISE

CUDDLE WITH A PUPPY

SOMEONE TO SIT WITH ME AND WATCH CRAPPY TV

TO BE LEFT TO SIT IN PEACE

Assemble your A-team

You're a strong, independent and super-capable human. So it can be very unnerving to ask for help and lean on your people. But you don't have to do this alone, nor should you, and helping each other is really what life is all about. This season is one when you can lean on those around you (and, trust me, they really want to help get you through this). Don't worry, in the ebbs and flows of life you'll get a chance to lift up the ones you love, further down the line. For now, though, surrender.

Who's on your team?

1 YOUR NEAREST AND DEAREST

One of the coolest things about a curveball is that you know instantly who are the most important people in your world. (It's a suboptimal yet super-efficient way to sort out the chaff from the real deal in your life. Ahh, silver linings.) I was so worried about being a burden – and it's not easy to be back in your childhood room at your parents' house, complete with fetching animal-print wallpaper (selected by my wholesome 15-year-old self) and an extensive pig collection to boot – but sometimes you just have to surrender and lean on your people.

You find when you go through a crisis that some people really step up and become super friends – they bring joy and delight into your day. Others fade away and are disappointing. Either way, it's actually a gift! You get to find out who really matters and who is always there for you, and you learn the value of your kind friends. As hard as it is, try not to get caught up in the people who disappoint you; it doesn't help you face the task ahead. Instead, focus on the excellent, awesome people and the lovely ways they are supporting you.

Remember that this is also a tough time for the people who love you (although you still get the gold medal of crappiness) and being a good support person is a delicate job. Inevitably, someone is going to say something silly, accidentally or because they don't know better or because they're human. Like the day after shaving off my hair, when my dad told me I looked like a monk, although he 'meant it in a really good way'. It was not taken in a 'really good way'! Poor Dad was mortified to upset me, but we can laugh about it now.

If someone says the wrong thing to you, try to breathe and keep calm before you respond. (Sure, you're allowed to spit the dummy here and there if you really need to, but it never makes you feel better. Trust me!)

If you don't have family or friends around and are feeling very isolated, I'm so sorry, that is really tough. Instead, try connecting with some of the excellent services and hotlines available. There is a list on pages 196–197.

- Who are the most important people in your world?
- Who do you need around you right now?
- Who might you need to see less of?

Having access to a professional counsellor during a challenging time can be incredibly beneficial and it's not a sign of weakness. **In fact, I'm going to say it's a must do!** It's a sign of strength to ask for guidance and support. Make sure it's someone you really click with. For example, the first psychologist I saw, well, let's just say we didn't exactly gel.

> *Psychologist: Why are you sad?*
>
> *Me: I'm three weeks into chemo, I feel like vomiting and today my hair started falling out.*
>
> *Psychologist: Why does that make you sad?*
>
> *Me: I don't want to be bald.*
>
> *Psychologist: Why?*
>
> *Me: (Thought bubble: Why the hell do you think? Are you a robot disguised as a human?)*
>
> Cue uncontrollable tears …

(Okay, if you're from a military background, that brutal line of inquiry might work for you, but I needed someone a little more Zen and soft around the edges, who would treat me like the delicate little millennial ball of cotton fluff that I am.)

I left bawling and determined never to see a psychologist ever again. It scared me off for a long time and, honestly, even though I was going through cancer I still wanted to PROVE to myself I was tough and didn't need help, and to show everyone how strong and awesome I was.

> Do you think you could benefit from speaking with a professional who has helped many others navigate what you're going through right now?

Please don't be like me! Sure, you might be able to wade your way through it, OR you could shortcut that process by speaking to someone who has helped hundreds of people go through what you are going through now. They might just have a better idea than you, who has dealt with this approximately zero times. A long way down the line I found someone with a style that was much more suited to me, who was gentle and sympathetic and got to know me before they started advising me. It was really helpful and I wish I'd done it sooner.

There are also great services and hotlines (see pages 196–197) for whatever you are experiencing that can be a helpful starting point if you don't know where to find a counsellor.

 NINJA TIP

PSYCHOLOGIST V PSYCHIATRIST

*A **psychologist** is a professional who has studied psychology at university, followed by further practical work and study. They will work in conjunction with your specialist or GP who can prescribe drugs if they are required.*

*A **psychiatrist** is a professional who has studied medicine, followed by psychiatry (they can prescribe drugs if you need them).*

There is nothing like the catharsis of chatting to someone who has been there, done that, got the T-shirt and emerged out the other side like a sparkly shiny legend. They truly get it and give you hope that, like them, one day you will be on the other side of this big old mess; be that a divorce, a health crisis or a gut-wrenching loss. So when you're ready, connect with someone you trust and respect who has already been through something similar to what you are experiencing. If you don't know anyone, ask friends to help you find someone.

My personal superhero was Luke, the lovely guy I'd worked with years before who had been through testicular cancer. Although we'd never really spoken of his experience before, I reached out to him and he became such an important person whom I knew I could call on any time to mull things over.

On my first call to Luke, I said to him, 'I don't want to know about chemo or treatment yet, I just want to have a chat and talk about how I'm feeling.' Everyone is different, some people might want to know every single bit of information possible. For me, I needed it to come in dribs and drabs. Remember, you're allowed to take in information at a pace that feels good to you. It's your crisis: you get to do what you want.

It's important to be really clear upfront about what you'd like to discuss and what areas might still be in the I'm-not-ready-for-this-yet camp.

④ SUPPORT GROUPS

There are so many online support groups these days that it should be easy to find one, but here's a word of warning: while these groups can be useful sources of information, they can also be a little overwhelming and daunting. There will be people on the full spectrum of suffering sharing their experiences in these groups, so you have no real control over the extent of what you are exposed to. You might hear stories of relapse in the case of illness, or people who have never been able to move on from the grief or trauma of their experience, and it can be very confronting. It might be handy to have a friend or family member enter the group for you and extract the information you require (my sister Molly did this for me) or just to test the waters for you before you dive on in.

- Who is in your A-team? Write down their names (and contact details) on a note on your phone or in your diary.
- Do you feel like you have the support you need?

- What else would make you feel secure and happy right now?
- Are there any other services you need to connect with? Can you ask someone in your A-team to help with that?

START A WHATSAPP GROUP

When a crisis first strikes, everyone will want to know what is happening and how they can help. Keeping everyone in the loop can become a full-time job. I recommend setting up a group on a communication platform such as WhatsApp or making a private Facebook page, and adding anyone who is reaching out, so you can easily update everyone at once.

You get to decide
what energy is
allowed around you.

Speak it out loud

No matter what is on your mind, if it's troubling you it's valid, even if you feel ridiculous for thinking certain thoughts. When you're going through a huge challenge, some pretty random ideas can pop up in your brain! I've found, however, that when you say things out loud it somehow takes their power away. Spoken out loud, worries can suddenly seem trivial, or you can't quite remember why they are upsetting you so much. No matter what is worrying you, find someone in your A-team and talk about it. Even if you think it sounds trivial, silly or self-absorbed. It can magically help 'expelliarmus' worries and take away their power. (I solemnly swear that will be the only Harry Potter reference in this book ... okay, I can't promise, but I'll try.)

Maybe you're dealing with something that feels too dark and scary to share. I remember in the early days of my diagnosis thinking that I should just die, because I didn't want to be a burden on everyone and the healthcare system. Perhaps my time was just up. When I look back now, I can't even believe I was having that thought! I spoke to my best friend Nikki, who is a doctor, about this fear. She helped me understand that we do so much to preserve life every day, that of course I deserved to be fixed and healed. But if I hadn't spoken it out loud, no one would have ever realised I was thinking such dark thoughts. You can't get help if no one but you knows what the problem is.

If you're going through a particularly nasty divorce or break-up you might think you'll never be loved again and you'll die alone (as if: you're so damn loveable there are heaps of people out there who will be busting to be with you once you get rid of that drain in your life). Or perhaps if you're experiencing grief because of the death of someone you love, you might be ruminating on never feeling happy again. No matter what it is, don't bottle it up, speak it out.

If you really don't feel ready to discuss it with someone else, journalling is a great way to help order your thoughts (more on this later). Put it into words with someone you feel safe with, and the power of these thoughts and words may start to dissipate.

Find someone you trust and talk it out.

What thoughts are running around in your head that would be good to talk about with someone you trust? Jot them down in a journal or notebook.

Put people at ease (because it will put you at ease)

As the person in the crisis, you may have to put people at ease by giving them some guidelines. I knew that the last thing I wanted was for people to feel like they were tiptoeing around me, or be so petrified of saying the wrong thing that they couldn't say anything at all. So from the get-go, I tried to be open and clear about what I was comfortable with and what I needed. I'd say to my friends:

'Just so you know, I'm probably going to cry at some point. If you need to cry, you cry, that's fine – you're not going to upset me any more than I already am.'

I could see people trying to 'hold it together' around me, but saying this to them seemed to release a pressure valve. I also said, 'You can ask me anything you want to know, I'm fine with that.' You might like to say, 'You can ask me how I'm feeling, but I don't want to talk about X right now.' Just lay down the framework for what you need. It might feel hard if you aren't used to it, but it will serve you better in the long run.

> What are you comfortable talking about right now? Who do you trust? What would make you feel safe and secure?

 NINJA TIP

CUT YOURSELF A LOT OF SLACK
When you're going through a crisis it's not the easiest time to make big decisions, but sometimes you have to. Know that you've made the best choice that you could under less-than-ideal circumstances, then let it go.

Be aware of the poisonous Ps

In the thick of my crisis, it really helped me to understand that there are three things that can affect our ability to cope. Renowned psychologist Martin Seligman created the concept of the three Ps: personalisation, pervasiveness and permanence. Getting a grasp of these little suckers while you navigate through can be really helpful.

1 PERSONALISATION

is the belief that you are at fault for everything that has happened. This can often be the case for survivors of rape; they blame themselves for their actions, for putting themselves in a vulnerable situation. We're good at making ourselves responsible for all kinds of things that are really not our fault. I blamed my lack of sleep and lifestyle for my lymphoma, but the truth is we don't know what causes it – and blaming myself certainly wasn't going to assist in my recovery.

2 PERVASIVENESS

is the belief that this event will affect all other aspects of your life. Early on in the experience of a trauma it can feel all-consuming. Understanding that your life will still be rich and lovely and exciting despite what has happened is really helpful. The trauma doesn't define you, it's just a part of your story. For me, yes, I had lymphoma, but I could still be a friend, a sister; I could still write and play music and do all manner of things that weren't affected by my illness, even at the worst times.

3 PERMANENCE

is the belief that you will ALWAYS feel this bad. However, even in the case of chronic illness, just because you feel really bad now doesn't mean it's always going to be like this. If you feel completely broken and don't know how you will ever get over it, remember that even the worst, most gut-wrenching pain or feelings are impermanent (as much as they suck at the time).

This is happening.

We wish it wasn't, but we can't go over it, we can't go under it, we have to bloody well go through it.

WELCOME TO THE SHIT SHOW. YOU'VE GOT FRONT-ROW SEATS!

I'm going to share a few things that really helped me when I was right in the thick of it and not feeling 100 per cent myself.

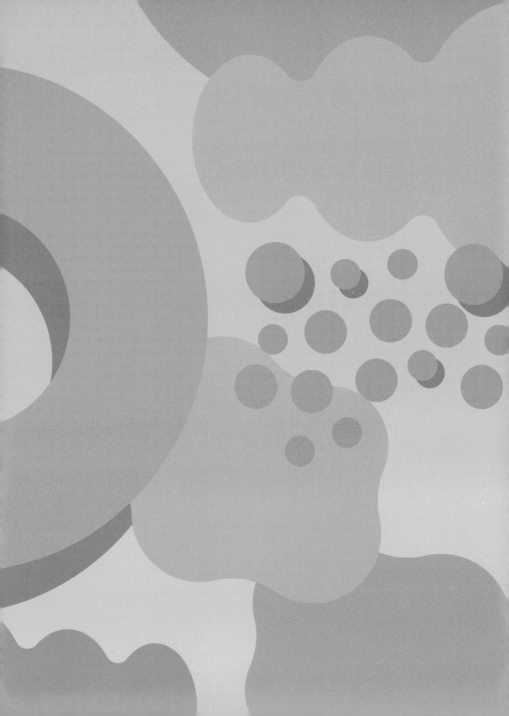

Ice Ice Baby

Twenty-four hours after I was diagnosed I found myself in another waiting room, this time at the IVF clinic, surrounded by young couples and soon-to-be-mums. Unlike the others in the waiting room, I sat there with my mum, holding her hand and thinking about my fertility properly for the first time in my life. Was I even fertile? If so, how many eggs did I have left? How do ovaries even work, exactly? Most importantly, would my babies be cute? It dawned on me that 31 was possibly a little late to be thinking about all this fertility stuff for the first time.

I'd just learned that when you go through chemo your ovaries can age by up to ten years – just what every gal wants. So if you have time, one option can be to freeze your eggs. As it turns out, when you have cancer they fast-track your IVF process and give you a large discount ... I mean, #worthit, right? (Amazingly the womb is not affected in the same way. Wombs are indestructible fortresses. No matter what is happening to the body, they're a badass bouncer that is like, 'Nah, you're not messing with my baby-making machine. Beat it, chemo!' How cool is the female body, seriously?)

Back in the waiting room, I was disappointed to find out I'd be seeing a male doctor and I felt a bit apprehensive. I shouldn't have been. The minute I walked in and met my doctor, Bill Ledger, his kind eyes and warm manner put me instantly at ease. He'd just come from seeing a 12-year-old who had recently been diagnosed with leukaemia and was looking at options for a tissue freeze. My scenario, by comparison, seemed like a walk in the park.

I sat down and Bill asked me warmly, 'So, Briony, how long have you known?'

My voice wobbled, but I tried to hold it together. 'Oh, about 24 hours,' I managed.

'You poor thing,' he said comfortingly. 'That's a lot to take in. Well today we're going to look at the options to freeze your eggs; it will be a great comfort to you when you go through treatment to know that your eggs are safely tucked away waiting for you on the other side of all this.

'Do you have a partner?' he asked.

I had been dating my then boyfriend for about 18 months. We certainly weren't at a point where we had discussed having children together, but a cancer diagnosis has a hell of a way of bringing on some major life conversations.

You know light, first-date kinda chats.

HEY BABE, DO YOU WANT YOUR EGGS SCRAMBLED, FRIED OR FERTILISED?

OH, JUST WONDERING IF YOU WANT TO FATHER MY POTENTIAL FUTURE CHILDREN THIS WEEK; SAY, THURSDAY?

HUH???

I decided to go ahead with the egg-freezing process, but it was a lot more complex than I realised. In my head, I thought it would involve sucking a few eggs out with some kind of device and off you go. I soon learned it's a little more complicated than that.

It involves hormone stimulation (in the form of daily injections) and multiple pelvic ultrasounds to check in on how the eggs are developing (nothing's as fun as a goo-covered rod being inserted into your vagina). When it's game time, you have a small procedure under anaesthetic where a needle is inserted through the vaginal wall into each ovary to extract the eggs. They snap-freeze those eggies and get them on ice and you pay an annual storage fee. The stats say that 12 eggs should give you a 50 per cent chance of having one baby ... but it's not guaranteed. And depending on how many eggs they manage to collect, you might need to go through multiple rounds. For me, I only had time to have one crack at this.

The day before I started chemotherapy, I had my procedure. My eggs had come along nicely and off we went to collect the fruits of my ovaries. Yes, it did feel very *Handmaid's Tale*.

After the procedure I woke up with a sticker on my hand with the number of eggs written on it and breathed a sigh of relief. The harvest had been fruitful, praise be! Bill came to congratulate me and wish me all the best for the next chapter. Act One was done: now it was time to get this chemo business knocked out.

Time to get this show on the road.

You can reframe just about anything

The toughest part for me (well, it made the top three shitty moments) was losing my hair. I won't beat around the bush: it was awful. Something my very wise younger sister Rhianna said at the time was that perhaps I could think, 'this means the medicine is working'. Now, you have to be careful giving advice to someone going through a challenging time. Unless you've been there and done that, or you're a professional, it's a risky move. My sister offered this very gently and it really helped me.

When my hair started falling out I was really distressed; I cried, I felt flat and low and so sad. I let myself feel it, but as each strand fell out I'd say to myself, 'The treatment is working. I'm a day closer to being on the other side of this.' It was a great lesson, that even in the most challenging moments, there is always a way to reframe what you are going through.

Instead of asking, 'Why is this happening to me?' it could be helpful to ask, 'What is this teaching me?' (Want to punch this page? No worries, let's move on.)

Sticks and stones will break your bones, but words can also be little pricks

When I was first diagnosed I never hated the lymphoma, because to do that would be to hate a part of myself. Instead, I tried to think lovingly of my lymph glands, which had just been doing their best but had gotten totally overwhelmed. Together we had to get out of this. Rather than hating my cancer, I instead thought about it passing through me.

Andy Puddicombe, the co-founder of one of the largest meditation programs in the world, headspace.com – which I highly recommend if you are going through a challenging time – has been through testicular cancer. He suggested that to use the language of fighting or hating cancer is to create tension or additional stress. (But if it works for you, go for it!)

LABEL WHAT YOU FEEL

This is a great tool to distance yourself from your emotions when they are overwhelming: rather than saying, 'I'm angry' or 'I'm anxious', instead try, 'This is anger' or 'This is anxiety'. It makes it more a temporary state of being and something that will pass rather than something that defines you. You're human, so of course you're going to experience these things, but don't embody it. Remember, it's just a feeling and it's just flowing through you.

Perhaps you're going through a break-up and you think, 'Why would anyone want to be with someone like me?' Stop those thoughts in their tracks! Instead you could think, 'I would not have been happy in the long term in that relationship. Better things are around the corner.'

Or if you're struggling to get up and feeling really exhausted each morning and you're thinking, 'I'm an idiot for staying up so late on my phone,' you could replace that thought with, 'It's okay if I'm feeling lonely and looking for connection, but I'll try to be better today and put my phone on airplane mode from 8 pm.' It's not helpful to be mean to yourself.

No matter what you are going through, be so careful with the words you direct towards yourself. If you wouldn't say it to a friend, don't say it to yourself.

I'm such an idiot ... *hey, don't speak about my friend like that!*

When you catch yourself thinking something mean of yourself, pause and ask, 'Is this a helpful thought? What is something else I could think? What am I doing really well right now?'

Force the LOLs and light

A divorce, a miscarriage, cancer, the loss of a loved one … what do these things have in common? They're not very funny – like, at all. When you're in the depths of despair it's really easy to forget to laugh, but adding lightness where possible and finding the opportunity to laugh is really good for the soul.

And those legendary scientists agree. Smiling and laughing releases endorphins, which are our body's own feel-good chemicals; it gives our immune systems a boost by reducing inflammation; and activates the release of serotonin, which is basically our body's own antidepressant. Laughter is a free wonder-drug with no nasty side effects. Even a fake smile can reduce your stress and boost your mood, so fake it till you make it!

Six weeks into chemotherapy I realised I hadn't really laughed at all, when my friend Jenna reminded me of the power of laughter. Cue Netflix comedy specials, and the laughs rolled in. Forced at first, but then they flowed. Do be sure to pull back on the intense TV shows and negative news stories. Be really careful about what you feed into your mind at this time. You know, a bit less of *The Handmaid's Tale* and a little more of *Bridget Jones's Diary*.

Research also suggests that any combination of movement, music and laughter is a potent prescription to boost your mood.

That's why I've taken to getting up most mornings and doing the world's daggiest dance party in my own bedroom to a bit of Taylor Swift, because T-Swizzle is the shizzle. Even though it's forced, your brain can't tell the difference. It will at least give you a little boost, and that's what you need and deserve.

> WATCH STAND-UP COMEDY (TRY OUT SOME NEW COMEDIANS ON STREAMING SERVICES).

> WATCH LIGHTHEARTED MOVIES.

> CALL YOUR FUNNIEST FRIEND AND CHAT.

> RECALL MOMENTS IN YOUR LIFE THAT HAVE MADE YOU LAUGH OUT LOUD.

> ORDER A SILLY OUTFIT FOR YOUR DOG.

> WHACK A PENCIL IN YOUR MOUTH AND FORCE YOURSELF TO SMILE.

> SEARCH YOUTUBE FOR 'PUPPIES + FUNNY' (WORKS EVERY TIME).

> FIND A COLLECTION OF REALLY FUNNY QUOTES OR JOKES AND SEND THEM TO FRIENDS.

> START A PUN WAR WITH A FRIEND WHO IS REALLY PUNNY.

Pick one thing from the list above that you will do today to make more space for laughter and light.

Journal your heart out

It's not an exaggeration to say that journalling was my greatest saviour throughout my treatment. Putting pen to paper morning after morning doesn't sound particularly game-changing, but it is. Okay, sure, the chemo drugs probably take line honours, but journalling was the rudder that calmed and navigated the journey for me.

I started a practice known as 'The Morning Pages'. It's a concept created by Julia Cameron in her book *The Artist's Way.* Basically, first thing in the morning every day you write out three pages. There is no right or wrong way to do this; there is no set topic or subject. It's basically just a giant brain dump on paper of whatever comes up for you.

By putting things into words, no matter whether it makes sense or not, you clear the thoughts from your mind so you can see your day with fresh eyes. Kind of like windscreen wipers for the soul. When you write at night or keep a diary, you might find that it tends to be more of a recollection of the day; however, if you write first thing in the morning, you are starting with a clean slate.

Nothing is off limits, you don't have to be positive or focus on anything in particular, but I find that if it's on my mind, out it comes. Some days my pages are a big old whinge, sometimes they're quite transcendent and I feel like a reincarnated prophet.

Journalling is particularly helpful during challenging times, and research shows that it not only gives a big boost to your memory and ability to be mindful, but it also strengthens the immune system, improves sleep, boosts confidence, makes you smarter and it may even help wounds heal faster!

Why? How? What is this sorcery? In a nutshell, writing is an organisational process, so it helps you make sense of trauma and process events. This improves your working memory and frees up your beautiful brain to get on with the million other tasks it has to do, rather than being stuck processing this experience.

When done daily, journalling starts to unlock you; you'll understand yourself better and see your life in greater clarity. I journalled religiously during my treatment. It felt healing and therapeutic, and there was also a sense of achievement to have started the day with a small goal knocked over. It gave me confidence that if I could stick to this, perhaps I could do anything. (You know, like write a book!) I also discovered it's very hard to lie on paper. I could tell myself all manner of things in my head, but when my pen touched paper, I found it virtually impossible to lie. I think this is why my morning pages became so powerful. It's hard to whinge about the same thing over and over and not think it might be time to make a change.

Buy a beautiful notepad and a pen you love ... it makes for a nice ritual each morning.

Set out your notepad and pen on a tidy desk the night before.

Don't try to 'write properly' or judge your writing or the thoughts – just let them flow.

Make sure you write the full three pages. You'll often find it takes two pages to warm up and you'll discover something very interesting on page three.

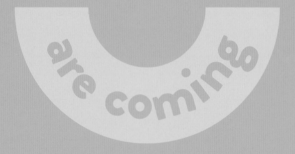

Just hang in there, legend.

This will make you more resilient

I know that in the Instagram age, being #grateful has gotten a bit of a bad rap. It seems so clichéd that it couldn't possibly work, right? But a gratitude practice became really important for me, especially on days I didn't feel like doing it.

Studies have shown that people who are more grateful experience less depression and are more resilient following traumatic events.

The simple pleasure of waking up and feeling good is a gift so many of us are given each day, but rarely take the time to stop and appreciate. I had a quote (often attributed to Marcus Aurelius) on the wall beside my bed and I'd read it every morning: 'When you arise in the morning, think about what a precious privilege it is to be alive: to think, to breathe, to love.'

It doesn't mean what you are going through isn't valid, but it helps to put it into perspective. When you start to look for the things you could be grateful for, you realise it's boundless. Your worst days may still be better than someone else's best-ever day.

So start looking at the magic, the gleaming beautiful moments, the richness you have right here, right now. You are more blessed than you know.

> Every night, ask yourself, 'What three things am I grateful for today?' Every morning when you wake up, try some grateful stretches. Move your body and start to wake it up while you think, 'What am I grateful for in my life?'

A LIST OF SURPRISING THINGS
I'VE FELT GRATEFUL FOR:

- My period. When it came back after chemotherapy, I cried. It was my body saying, 'We are well enough to support a life.' Bloody hell, I never thought I'd feel appreciative of my period! (The matter of finding someone to create a life with is a whole other affair.)

- Eyebrows! I used to really bemoan my uneven brows, but when they were gone completely I thought if they grew back I would never, ever, ever complain about them again. I'd love them like crazy! Even though they are slightly non-symmetrical.

- Waking up and feeling well. Nothing more, just thinking, 'I don't feel nauseous: this is a great day!'

- Having access to chemotherapy. It's not something you'd pick off the menu at a day spa, but I felt lucky my body was able to have it and lucky to live in a country that gave me access to world-class free medical care. (In America, the number-one cause of bankruptcy is healthcare bills.*) Looking after every person when they are most vulnerable is, I believe, one of the most important components of a caring, functional society.

- My dog. Okay, that's not really surprising: he was ridiculously cute and my constant companion through chemo. He was glued to my side and it was delightful.

Create the movie trailer of your life

If you could create a trailer of all the good bits of your life and cut it together and watch it each day, how amazing would that be? Our life is filled with extraordinary moments, big and little, and it's nice to relive them.

Well, you can. This is a great technique that I found handy to supercharge my gratitude. Rather than just listing all the things you are grateful for – your health, your family, your dog, this sunshiny day – simply close your eyes and go back to moments in your life that have been wonderful. They may be small moments or really key life events, but go back and relive them in your mind. Remember what it looked like, how you felt, who was there, how it smelt. Go back and be in that moment. Then add another memory, and another.

What you end up with is this kick-arse highlights reel of all of the most sublime moments of your life. You can replay it in the theatre of your mind whenever you like, and you're the star of the show.

 Keep an album on your phone of screenshots of lovely messages, quotes, photos and moments. You can flick through it when you need a little pep up!

SCENES FOR YOUR LIFE MOVIE

> BEAUTIFUL MEMORIES OF
> THOSE YOU LOVE

> THINGS YOU'VE DONE WITH
> PEOPLE YOU REALLY LOVE

> BIG ACCOMPLISHMENTS

> NICE THINGS PEOPLE
> HAVE DONE FOR YOU

> MOMENTS YOU'VE FELT
> TOTALLY EXHILARATED

> YOUR FAVOURITE MEALS
> AND WHERE YOU'VE
> HAD THEM

> FALLING IN LOVE

> TIME SPENT IN NATURE

> A TIME YOU FELT
> REALLY LOVED

> YOUR BEST CHILDHOOD
> ACHIEVEMENT

> A TIME YOU WERE MOST
> PROUD OF YOURSELF

> TRAVEL, CAMPING,
> ADVENTURES

> BEAUTIFUL SIGHTS
> YOU'VE SEEN

> WHEN YOU LAUGHED
> TILL IT HURT

> SOMETHING FUNNY
> A PET DID

Now get editing.

Can you create a trailer
of your life and replay it
weekly? Take a moment
to relive the most amazing
memories of your life.

If I have to do
this anyway,
how can I make
it more fun?

You can't polish a turd, but you can roll it in glitter

In the aftermath of chemo, I really didn't enjoy having short hair. Mum and I got thinking about how we could make this experience of recovery and having short hair more fun. We came up with the idea to find celebrities and film characters who had shaved heads and do photo re-creations. Think Charlize Theron looking badass in *Mad Max: Fury Road*, or Demi Moore as G.I. Jane.

My mum sourced costumes and props from things we had lying around the house, and then we'd find a backdrop in the house or garden to replicate the picture. Mum was Executive Producer as well as head of the camera department and lighting, costumes, props. My sister Molly helped with make-up.

The point is that there is always a way to make something more fun than it is, such as wearing bright lippy to chemo appointments, or going to get pedicures with your mates (including the blokes). When I was feeling down I'd ask, 'If I have to do this anyway, how can I make it more fun?' Sure it doesn't always work: some days you just want to get through it without the added burden of also being the court jester.

But I think it's a good question to ask in life generally, not just when you're dealing with a crisis.

> Ask yourself, how can I make this more fun, or at least a bit less crap?

Get handsy

It's nice to get out of your head and use your hands. So many of the things I enjoy are all related to being stuck in my head, such as reading non-fiction, writing, listening to TED Talks and watching documentaries. They don't really give your head any downtime.

Then my friend Francine brought me a loom and a big bag of coloured wool and spent time teaching me how to use it (such an excellent and thoughtful gift idea). It was lovely to create nice handmade gifts for friends' babies and get fully immersed in a creative activity.

Working with our hands has been shown to relieve stress and help us work through our problems. It allows our brains some time out from being very clever and serious, so they can just chill out while we get busy in the garden.

So why not have a crafternoon?

* I HIGHLY RECOMMEND THE UKULELE - IT'S CHEAP, EASY AND BOPPY.

IS THERE A HANDS-ON ACTIVITY YOU'VE ALWAYS WANTED TO TRY?

CLAY MODELLING OR POTTERY

LEARN A CARD TRICK

KONMARI YOUR CUPBOARDS

PAINTING

GARDENING

KNITTING

LEARNING A MUSICAL INSTRUMENT*

SCRAPBOOKING

WOODWORK

HOME-BREWING

WREATH-MAKING

BAKING

THERE'S LIGHT AT THE END OF THE TUNNEL

Good days are coming, so here are a few things
to consider as you catch your breath.

The closest I'll come to being a Hogwarts student

One of the most physically painful times through the whole experience of treatment for me was in my second round of chemotherapy, when I had to have injections to help replenish my bone marrow. It was excruciating.

The only way I can describe it is that it felt like each one of my bones was screaming. Or, for the Harry Potter fans among us, the way it must have felt when Harry was given a magic potion to regrow every bone in his arm after a particularly bad Quidditch accident. (Just like that, except all over my body and sadly without any Quidditch, magic or butterbeer.)

For two days I was in such blinding pain that I was in and out of consciousness. It was the most pain I've ever experienced in my life. This was getting tough and I wasn't even halfway through chemotherapy yet. I was now bald, feeling pretty nauseous and certainly not at my most glamorous. The following week I had my check-up at the hospital and a PET scan to see how things were progressing. I was worried: I felt so bad that I didn't think the chemo had even touched the sides. My support crew (Mum, Dad and Molly) came to the hospital with me to receive the results.

We sat down with my specialist, the brilliant Dr Tara Cochrane.

'You're in remission,' she stated.

I inhaled sharply.

'What exactly does that mean?' I asked cautiously.

'It means we can't see the cancer anywhere in your body.'

It was nearly as much of a shock as finding out that I had lymphoma in the first place. I was stunned but ecstatic, and couldn't help the tears welling up.

We left the hospital, stopped in the sunshine on the way out and held each other tight. Mum – who had held it together until then and had never once lost it in front of me – sobbed, as though she could finally let it out.

Anyone walking past would have thought that we had just received some really bad news. We went for lunch once more by the sea to celebrate the win and to take in this glorious, ordinary, extraordinary day.

I was not out of the woods yet, but I had come up and taken a giant breath of air.

It was a great reminder that things can be bad and getting better at the same time.

Perhaps you've seen a glimmer, a flicker of hope that things aren't always going to be so hard. You've had a positive moment or a day you've felt better than usual. You've had a laugh with a friend and momentarily forgotten about what else is happening. There is a light at the end of the tunnel, and you're quite confident it isn't a train.

Take in all the glorious magic around you

One of the greatest joys of my experience of cancer was slowing down and having time to properly appreciate the beautiful small details of life. In a rush to achieve and do 'important things', we forget that big lives are made up of little moments, and if we're not careful we might just miss our whole life while we are scrambling to think about the next moment. I loved the process of actually having the time and patience to take in more of life.

It's the little moments: belly laughs with friends, steam rising from a morning cuppa, receiving a letter in the mail, taking in a sunset, being in the presence of those who love you. It sounds trite, but I REALLY mean it. I'm so much better at savouring these moments now than I used to be.

I find myself far more often in a state of awe at the world around me, particularly the natural world. Have you ever just sat and watched a spider build a web? It's actually mind-blowing to think this tiny creature could make an invisible yet incredibly strong home that can catch and store food and that glistens in the sunlight. (I am still scared of spiders, but I can appreciate the beauty in what they do.) Or just looking up at the night sky, and the moon and the stars will take your breath away. There's a spectacular show being put on and it's a million times more dazzling than anything you'll find on your phone or on Netflix.

Once you begin to slow down and really look, you start to see the world in a whole new light. There is magic all around us; we just have to look for it.

What little moments have you enjoyed this week?

Happy hacks and other mood boosters

SING IN THE MORNING

It's really good for the soul

PLANT A SMALL GARDEN

or tend to some herbs and potted plants if you don't have much space

LEARN SOMETHING NEW

Do a course, watch a talk, listen to a podcast, master a new skill

HAVE CUDDLES AND PATS WITH A PET

If you don't have one, accost someone else's

PLANT SOME SPROUTS OR BEAN SHOOTS

Grow plants that you can nurture (and then eat)

KEEP YOUR PHONE OUT OF YOUR ROOM AT NIGHT!

(I know you need an alarm clock, so just buy an alarm clock)

There is
magic all
around us.

We just have
to look for it.

Setting up mindful moments

My mind runs at a million miles an hour, so meditation is something I've always struggled with (although I still try most days). I understand its value and I'm getting better at it; however, something I've found really achievable and simple is to take a few 'mindful moments' each day. It's a helpful way to begin. The plan is to set up five to ten mindful moments in a day that can be built into your routine.

A mindful shower

When I'm in the shower, I'm usually thinking of approximately 327,439 other things. So I try to take a few moments to feel the water landing on my skin, sense the warmth, notice what every little drop looks like as it falls from the showerhead and how pretty the droplets are in the light. I take a deep breath and inhale the aroma of the soap or shampoo. Such richness in one small morning experience that I would normally miss. It helps me slow down and feel calm.

Mindfully eating

When I'm eating I'm prone to scoff my food down while I check my phone or get a quick TikTok hit. I realised that it had been a long time since I truly stopped and enjoyed my food. I started to actually smell the food I was eating; I'd take in the colours on the plate and the shapes and sizes of the different things I was about to bite into. I try to actually think about the flavour and textures inside my mouth: how they feel on my tongue. Even taking in the details of a piece of fruit can be quite an amazing experience.

Some other mindful moments

- Listen to the sounds around you. Are they close by or far away? Indoors or outdoors?

- As you walk, notice the way your feet feel inside your shoes and how it feels as the weight of your body transfers from the heel to the ball of your foot with each step.

- List five things around you right now that you can see, hear, smell and touch.

- When you brush your teeth, take a moment to feel the textures and flavours in your mouth and the sensation of the brush moving against your teeth.

- Lie on your back in the park and look at the sky. Notice details, shapes and colours.

- Watch an insect or animal going about its day.

Finding time for these small pockets of calm can really enrich your day, make it feel more expansive and help you to slow down and add more joy to your life.

Set up a little reminder on your phone for mindful moments throughout the day. Start with just one a day and then build up. It might seem counterintuitive to use your phone for this, but it's just to get you into the habit.

Look for silver linings

In the years leading up to my diagnosis, I would meet my dear friend Tim every Wednesday morning and we would do the famous Bondi to Bronte coastal walk in Sydney. It became our weekly therapy. With the warm sun shining down on us and the ocean glistening like diamonds, it was the most stunning backdrop for pondering the big questions, to top up the soul and start the day.

One particular morning it was overcast, windy and spitting rain. I groaned; I'd much prefer to be in bed, bemoaning the horrid morning. I crossed my arms and braced myself against the 'awful' weather. We started walking and I soon realised that, where normally the path would be crowded with hundreds of others, we had it and the ocean all to ourselves. In a busy city like Sydney, that was a rare treat. The overcast sky had created a dramatic backdrop of colours (the sparkling aqua water had been replaced with deep rich blues, greens and greys). And far away on the horizon a small patch of sun was peeking through the clouds and sending down sunbeams onto the glimmering ocean. I realised it wasn't ghastly after all; in fact, it was spectacularly beautiful when I stopped for a moment and appreciated it for what it was, not what I wanted it to be.

Look, I do still hate being cold, and walking in the rain will never be my first choice, but it was a great reminder that there is so often a silver lining. And if you can't see or sense a silver lining right now, that's fine too. You don't have to force it. Sometimes there just isn't one and that's okay.

Some silver linings

Being physically incapacitated... having time to appreciate the little things.

Not hearing from my friends... realising who was really worth my time and energy.

A relationship breaking up... understanding that this wouldn't have lasted anyway. What a gift to have found out now and not many years down the track.

Having to move away from my 'life'... being able to reconnect with my family and friends whom I adore.

Not being able to work... slowing down and thinking about what really matters and what I actually want to do with my life.

Having my looks and 'identity' completely changed... developing new-found confidence in myself that isn't linked to my physical appearance.

This is just one day

Whatever happens today, remember
that it's just one day in your life.
If it didn't pan out today, that's okay.

The world is still a wonderful place.
Someone's kid walked for the first time today,
someone fell in love, there is kindness everywhere
and places for you still to see and wonderful people
for you still to meet.

If it's not your day today, your day is coming.
Tomorrow is a clean slate. Let yourself off the hook.
Don't overthink it too much.
A night's rest will recharge your battery and
you can start again tomorrow.

In your beautiful, rich, expansive life,
this is just one little blip.

Your life

this
moment

This won't break you, and it just might make you.

Be more tree

After I found out I was in remission, I had an enormous blood clot, which meant I needed another six weeks of regular tests and check-ups. Then there was a break-up; things just kept hitting me in waves. I think trees are a good metaphor for how I got through.

When it's blowing a gale, look at the treetops: do they stand rigid against the storm? No. If they did they would snap in half. Instead they sway, bend and move with it, while staying firmly rooted in the ground. A dear friend and mentor told me that as he has navigated the trickier seasons of life this idea has made all the difference: sometimes in life you have to be a bit bendy.

The storm will eventually pass. Yes, you may feel rattled and have shaken off some leaves in the process, but there are blue skies above those clouds. So when it's all feeling a bit rough and you don't think you can take any more, remember to channel your inner tree and sway with the wind.

HOW TO BE MORE TREE

> BE BENDY

> GROW STRONG ROOTS WHILE THE WEATHER IS FINE

> STAND TALL – IT MAKES YOU FEEL BETTER

> GET PLENTY OF WATER

> NURTURE THOSE AROUND YOU

> ALWAYS KEEP GROWING

> REALISE THAT YOU CAN'T BLOOM ALL YEAR ROUND

Think about what you're looking forward to

Having something to look forward to beyond the crisis can be really helpful. It might be something small, such as going for nature walks or taking up a hobby, or something bigger, such as going on a special trip or starting a new project or course. Write it down and put it somewhere you can see it, or create a vision board of the things you are looking forward to. These can help give you a glimmering light at the end of the tunnel.

I created a giant photo wall of all my favourite people, fun memories and helpful quotes that I could look at every day to remind myself of all the goodness in my life. Then I created one with images of all of places I'd like to visit in the future. I also wrote out a list of things I was pumped to do after treatment. One of those things was going to visit my little sister overseas. That became a beacon that I could look towards when inevitable setbacks took place.

Remember that so often it is hardships and awful situations that propel us on to great things. It can be hard to feel that when you're in the thick of it and it's all a bit foggy. Often the worst things that happen to us can put us on track to super-awesome people, relationships and journeys that would not have happened otherwise. For now, just keep plodding through and remember that this won't break you; it might just make you.

> **What are you looking forward to once you're through this sticky bit?**

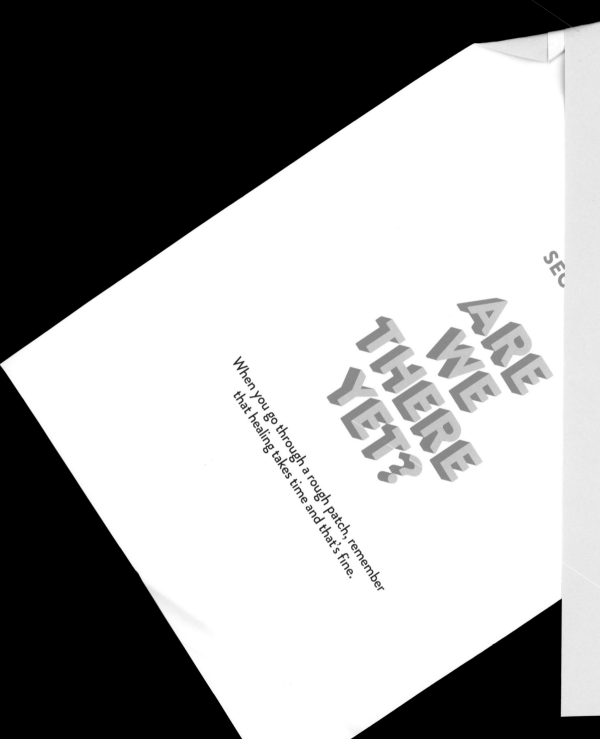

ARE
WE
THERE
YET?

SEC...

When you go through a rough patch, remember that healing takes time and that's fine.

The little apple seed

While I was having chemo, I bit into an apple and found a seed that had split open and begun to sprout. I placed the seed on a little bit of cotton wool in water, tended to it daily and slowly watched it grow as my hair and strength grew, too.

But, gosh, it took a while to grow. Two years later, it's still not a big tree bearing delicious apples (much to my surprise). It's a small and vulnerable little sapling that lives in a pot on a sunny ledge outside the kitchen at my parents' house, where they tend to it daily. It's had periods where it lost all of its leaves, and Mum has brought it back from the brink a few times, with lots of love and seaweed emulsion.

It reminds me a lot of my healing and recovery (minus the seaweed emulsion). The whole process has taken sooo much longer than I would have hoped, and I've had to finally accept that my life needs to adjust to a different pace. And that's okay: some things cannot be rushed. It's a much more sustainable way to live and is full of richness in other ways. As Ralph Waldo Emerson wrote, 'Adopt the pace of nature. Her secret is patience.'

When you go through a relationship breakdown, a health crisis or the loss of something or someone you love, the slow pace of healing can be seriously frustrating. I know I wanted so desperately to 'get back to normal'. You can feel really disappointed in yourself when you're still not over a heartbreak years down the track, or your health is still wobbly. It takes time. And I've found that the more I've pushed, the slower my recovery has been.

Remember that no matter what you're going through, you can start something new: plant a seed, an idea, make a change and watch it grow. I'm still learning how to be patient and move through the world at a new pace and energy. I've crashed and burned so many times on the way to recovery. But I'm learning to give myself the space I need to recover, physically, emotionally and spiritually. I love my life and I'm grateful for every day I get to live and grow.

NINJA TIP *Healing takes time. Pace yourself: on days when you feel bad, do a little more than you think you can; on days you feel great, do a little less than you are capable of. This will keep your momentum going.*

SLEEP + GOOD FOOD + MEDITATION +

LOTS OF LOVE FOR YOURSELF + TIME = HEALING

Your body wants to heal

A few months after I finished chemotherapy, I decided that I'd earned a holiday (right?), so I went to see my sister in London. It felt like a big step after my treatment. Luckily, on the plane I sat beside a woman named Alice, who had a warm smile and splendid red hair (my favourite: I was obsessed with *Anne of Green Gables* as a kid). It was as if the universe had sent me someone whom I needed at that time: Alice had a background as a physiotherapist at the Peter MacCallum Cancer Centre and she told me a powerful thing that has stayed with me ever since:

Remember, your body wants to heal.

It was such a mind shift for me.

Isn't it funny how we see the process of recovery as an annoying thing that comes between us and a normal life? We just want to fast-forward through it. Even the language around recovery is so rushed! 'Wishing you a SPEEDY recovery'; 'You'll smash this'; 'You'll be on your feet in no time'.

I get it: it's super frustrating when you just want to live your life. But I realise now that healing cannot be rushed. (Trust me, I tried and it really does not work!) We need to treat our bodies with love and kindness even when it feels like they have let us down. In the case of emotional pain, it is also going to take time.

Have patience with your soul, it needs some time and space.

Think of three ways you can give your body and heart the support it needs to heal itself; for example, drinking more water, stretching daily or getting more sleep. Even the very smallest incremental changes you make can all add up.

What is good for you is not good for me

Our bodies are all different and move at different paces. Look at how two bodies respond to the same virus or bug: some people have almost no symptoms at all, while others might become terribly unwell. Don't compare your experience to the speed at which others move about in the world or recover. Just like comparing yourself to that shiny, tanned, impossibly beautiful Instagram model with the perfect house/teeth/boyfriend/two-piece activewear set/dog, it doesn't make you feel all that good.

Something that is good for someone else is not necessarily good for you. Things that others get away with may not work for you. (Some of my friends can go on a three-day bender and seemingly never get sick, but that's not me!) Love your body, listen to your body and give it what it needs.

Remember, your body is the only place you have to live and it's doing its very best.

It's on your side and it wants to heal.

How to steady yourself when you're feeling wobbly

Once I was out of the washing machine of chemo, I thought it would all be smooth sailing as I returned to my old life, that the worst had been done and dealt with. But, for me, that is when it became the hardest emotionally. After any major trauma, once the 'doing' has been done, you have time to reflect and try to make sense of it all, and work out what you want to do next.

I'd moved back into my share house in Sydney, but my friends had since moved out; I had really short hair for the first time in my life and looked radically different; I'd been through a relationship break-up and was trying to sprint back into my old life, but I wasn't sure I fit anymore and I just didn't feel myself. I felt exhausted and kept wearing myself out, which would make me feel worse. I couldn't quite see the end in sight, and I wondered if this was how I'd always feel now? How long would this exhaustion last?

I steadied myself with this little phrase that I wrote out on a small piece of orange paper and left on my bedside table. I wrote a vision of where I wanted to get to and how I wanted to feel. I read it most days, especially when I was feeling unsettled or dismayed. It said:

YOU'RE GOING TO GET THROUGH THIS, AND YOU'RE GOING TO COME BACK BRIGHTER AND SHINIER AND STRONGER AND WISER AND MORE GORGEOUS THAN EVER BEFORE.

As I read it over and over again, I started to believe it. And slowly, very slowly, I started to feel better, more settled and calm.

Focus on the things that feel good

We spend so much time focusing on the negatives and what we'd like to improve. Gosh, we're really just so mean to our dear little selves sometimes, aren't we?

I had some photos taken a few weeks before my diagnosis and I remember thinking that my hair was sitting weirdly, I had a wonky smile and I didn't like my arms. A few months later when I had no hair and eyebrows, I looked at those photos and thought, 'Oh my goodness, I was more gorgeous than I ever realised.' What if we just got over ourselves and obsessed about all the cool things our bodies allow us to do?

A yoga teacher once told me not to focus on the areas that felt painful and sore during practice, but to think about all the parts that felt really good. What a shift! It's so easy to fixate on the pain, especially when it's sitting there yelling at the top of its lungs and poking you for attention.

But it's worth remembering today, right here and right now, you are younger than you will ever be again. And you are more awesome than you realise.

> WHAT IS YOUR FAVOURITE PART OF YOUR BODY?

> WHAT'S SOMETHING YOU LOVE DOING THAT YOUR BODY ALLOWS YOU TO DO?

> WHAT FEELS REALLY GOOD RIGHT NOW?

Pick something you like about your body and focus on that.

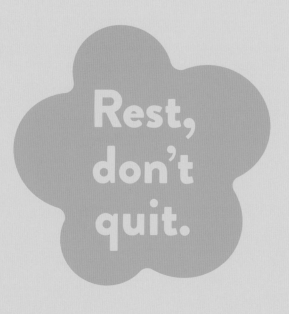

Rest,
don't
quit.

Remember,
you're awesome,
but you're also
exhausted.

Make it about someone else

Living is giving. And while doing good is nice, it also makes us feel better (win–win). For me, doing good looked like helping others along who had just started their cancer journey, people who had reached out to me on social media. I'd catch up IRL (in real life) with them and try to give them encouragement and hope. It took the focus off me and my recovery and it felt so good to give others help in really practical ways. Many strong friendships have formed from this.

A few months out of chemo, I was struggling a fair bit emotionally. My mother gently suggested it was time for me to start doing more for other people. She was right. So I reached out to an organisation to help do some tutoring with students at a school nearby who needed the extra support. I love doing it every week and it gives me such a boost, knowing I'm helping in some small way. It's funny but true that often when you help others you end up helping yourself more.

Some ideas for helping others

- Send someone you love a message to say that you love them and you are grateful to have them.

- Bake a friend some treats and drop them over.

- You could drop a note to an elderly neighbour or even go and say hi.

- Offer to babysit someone's children to give them a night off, or look after someone's pets.

- Help your parents clean up their computer (they will think you are a tech oracle from the future).

Let yourself off the hook

Sometimes we really just need to lighten up and give ourselves a break. When you're feeling crap, some days, if you get up, make your bed and get through the day then that is enough. Expect less of yourself when you're in recovery mode. Because you really have one major job and that is to recover (and that really is a full-time job).

When I was recovering, I had two simple questions that I wrote up on my wall. They were the only things I had to accomplish each day.

How are you ... *calming your mind today?*

How are you ... *strengthening your body today?*

So if I did a gentle walk and a meditation then – BINGO – that was a successful day, no more questions asked! And if I didn't do it, that was okay too.

Know that by being gentle and kind to yourself and treating yourself like the precious little gem you are, you will become STRONGER in time.

What is the one thing you want to focus on daily while you recover?

What to do if you're feeling flat

Here's my little checklist. You might like to make your own version or adapt this.

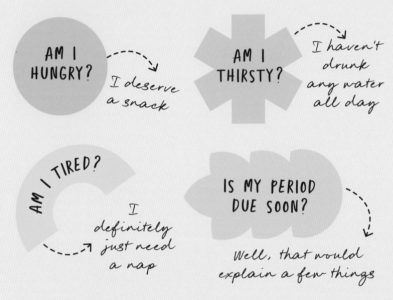

I don't know why, as a full-grown lady, my period still takes me by surprise – like every month, without fail, I'm totally unaware. (What ... again???) But if you're getting sad or overly emotional about something, just first ask, 'Is my period due soon?' then go ahead and cry and feel your feels. It can sometimes be good for context to know that it might just be exacerbating things a little.

I've realised that a nap or a good laugh are basically the human version of turning the computer off and on again. Doesn't work every time but, quite often, it's pretty good advice.

If that doesn't solve the problem, maybe:

- Have a bath.
- Have a nap or, if you can't nap, lie down and listen to a podcast.
- Go for a walk in the park and listen to music that makes you feel nice.
- Do something with your hands.
- Breathe in for four counts, hold for four and breathe out for six counts (and repeat).

- Keep a journal of your moods and feelings so you can discover any patterns.
- Call a friend.
- Do something for someone else.
- Write a letter or send a text to someone you love.
- Watch some comedy.
- Give yourself the day off: it's just one day.

It's okay to be flat lemonade

My mum says this to me when she sees me using up too much energy.
I've always been a bubbly character and that's how I love being with my friends and people I meet. But sometimes you just don't have the energy for that and you have to rein yourself in a little.
Don't dig into your reserves.
You're still lovable just as you are, without the bubbles for now.
It's okay to be flat lemonade.

You might not know what you want to do next, and that's fine

When the storm has passed and the dust has settled, here's a little word of warning: life may never return to 'normal'. Your experience may have stretched you in ways you would not have expected and given you a completely different view of life; of its fragility, of its uncertainty and of its beauty and wonder. You may find your work no longer provides you with the satisfaction or meaning you crave, or perhaps some of your relationships no longer serve you. This isn't a bad thing: it means you have grown and you are moving on to richer, more exciting things that light you up and give you more meaning. It can, however, be unnerving.

I've spent a lot of time trying to get my life 'back on track'. I realise that going off track is okay.

You can use up an immense amount of energy trying to force yourself back into your old life.

Or you can step forward into the rich future that is ahead.

I want you to know that after a major life curveball, it is so normal to feel completely confused and lost. You're not losing the plot, you are NORMAL. Everything you've known has just been flipped upside down. Once you're through the 'business' of dealing with the trauma – completing chemotherapy, finalising the separation, organising a funeral – it can be harder in a whole other way. Because now you have time to think and reflect and really question what you are doing with your precious time on Earth and what you want to do next. These aren't exactly simple questions!

DO NOT FRET. We all feel like this. Instead, try to have patience, roll with it, welcome the questions and thoughts and know that you don't have to make any hard-and-fast decisions straight away. Give yourself time to process the events and know that what you are feeling is TOTALLY NORMAL and TOTALLY VALID.

Have patience as you recover, taking it one step at a time. Enjoy the moments you are living right now, the questions, the discoveries and the evolution of your soul.

Things that can help you figure out the next chapter:

- Journalling regularly
- Counselling from someone you connect with
- Spending time in nature
- Meditating daily

- Being patient
- Understanding this is all part of the process
- Talking it through with loved ones*

If you're a woman this comes naturally – it's called brunch – but if you're a bloke you might need to get better at asking for help and sharing your vulnerability. No one can help you if they don't know there is a problem.

It's never too late to start

When you've had time to rebuild, regain your strength and put on your oxygen mask, you may decide that you want to try something totally new. Perhaps you've felt like it's too late for you to change your life. You're locked in. You picked your direction some years ago and now you're stuck with that decision. I'm telling you now, that is absolute bullshit. It pains me so much when I hear people talk about how they hate their lives and their jobs: it's the greatest tragedy; someone tortured by their daily existence. It is NEVER too late to start again.

The world is full of glittering examples of people who have done extraordinary things later in life. Vera Wang, the world-famous fashion designer, didn't create her first dress until she was 40. Television chef Julia Child didn't even learn to cook until she was 36 years of age and didn't begin teaching until she was nearly 40. Then, on the extreme end of the spectrum, there's my spirit animal, Anna Mary Robertson Moses, a prolific and acclaimed folk artist who didn't start painting until she was 78! She exhibited internationally all through her nineties and continued painting until a few months before her death at the age of 101. What a lady! But it's not all about fame and glory. I use these examples simply to show that remarkable things can happen when we follow whatever lights us up; when you go towards the things that make your soul happy and give you purpose and comfort and momentum.

> What weekly activities could you introduce into your life to bring more joy and creativity?

So, please, I beg you from the bottom of my heart: start. Start small if you like. You don't have to throw it all in and blow up your life to start experimenting with things that bring you joy. What are the things your soul has always yearned for? To paint? To write poetry or to walk the Camino? Maybe you could attend a weekly art class, or make space once a week to write some poetry, or start doing some nearby walks. Perhaps it's learning about a new career that has fascinated you or learning a musical instrument. The biggest regrets in life will be the things you never did. There is no rush, you have time. But when you're ready, plant your little apple seed.

If you're tired, rest, don't quit

When you're feeling awful or flat, it's so easy to start feeling negative or thinking about giving up completely.

You feel like your ambitions are drying up. Sometimes even simple things like getting groceries and cooking meals, or getting dressed and out the door on time can feel like mammoth never-ending tasks. I've had times when I've thought, I'll never want to work again.

But remember, you just need to rest and take it in your stride. If you have children or other responsibilities that you can't put aside, are there family and friends you can turn to and ask for more support?

Remember, you're not lazy and useless, you're exhausted and need to rest.

SOME WORDS OF WISDOM FROM A FRIEND

I asked for advice from a few special friends when I got sick. My friend Jenna offered me such valuable guidance and wisdom that I wanted to share it with you.

Jenna has been managing chronic fatigue syndrome for the past decade and a half, which developed after she contracted a mystery tropical illness at 23 years of age.

Jenna is sunshine in human form: I also think there's a 99 per cent chance she's magical. I mean, get this: she lives in the rainforest, rears baby wildlife (sugar gliders, wallaby joeys and so on), runs swimming-with-whales expeditions and owns an organic tropical fruit ice-cream company that makes exquisite flavours such as jackfruit gelato and passionfruit sorbet (see, pure magic). But dear Jenna has been navigating the murky waters of living with, at times debilitating, chronic fatigue. So what do you do when you are faced with something that isn't just going to be over at some clear future date? Jenna is a wealth of knowledge about creating a life of meaning despite your circumstances. So I'm going to hand these next pages over to her, so she can share with you the same wisdom that most helped me.

To follow Jenna's adventures, and for a daily hit of wildlife cuteness, you can find her and the fur babies she raises on Instagram: @wild.life.rescue.

Jenna's story

At 23 I was travelling through the South Pacific – a trip that was meant to be a footnote in my life's story, but instead became the backdrop – when I was struck down with a debilitating virus. I became a fixture in the waiting rooms of GPs, specialists, pathology labs and hospitals, getting every test under the sun. I desperately clung to the hope of a diagnosis and treatment plan that would enable me to resume the life I loved as an energetic and adventure-seeking marine biologist. But the fabled magic pill never appeared and, eventually, I was told I had chronic fatigue syndrome (CFS): a complex and debilitating multisystem disease. There is no cure.

This was the medical equivalent of being the last kid picked in handball. Unlike most illnesses, CFS is often determined by the elimination of other potential candidate diseases, instead of any definitive test ('… and then there was one'). Some people recover from this disease after a few years, some after a few decades, some never. And the kicker is there is no way of telling which camp you are going to be in. So far, I am at the 14-year mark.

My degree of disability has ranged in severity from being bed-bound and needing help with the most basic tasks (you don't know true romance until your partner has carried you to and from the loo) to being moderately functional, where people I know casually don't even know there is anything wrong. Every day is a balancing act. So, what do you do when the usual platitudes of 'this shall pass' and 'you can beat this' don't apply? You face your fear and do a deep dive into yourself.

Living with chronic illness is complex and I certainly don't have all the answers, but I can share the strategies and mindsets that have helped me through the most difficult times. I hope they serve as a source of comfort and guidance as you navigate your own journey.

FOCUS ON ABUNDANCE

I find it a helpful practice, particularly when I'm feeling down, to make a conscious effort to switch my perspective from one of scarcity (what you have lost) to one of abundance (what you have gained). Approaching a challenging circumstance as an 'opportunity' rather than a 'threat' can help shift your focus towards attaining something rather than losing it.

One of the many things you may have been gifted with in your new situation is time. A precious commodity with which to explore your interests. I encourage you to take this opportunity to feed your curiosity.

Always been fascinated by calligraphy? Watch videos and learn the craft. Never got around to reading the classics? Lose yourself in *The Great Gatsby* or listen to an audio book of *War and Peace*. Even just listening to an engaging podcast or TED Talk can change what would otherwise have felt like a wasted 'sick day' into one where you have learned something new, and therefore grown in some way.

Shifting your mindset from scarcity to abundance can also help in other areas of life. During the writing of this book my beloved father unexpectedly passed away. To help deal with the grief, I have purposefully shifted my focus from one of overwhelming loss to one of abundance: I'm grateful for the many memories, experiences, lessons and laughter we shared. Of course, there are times when I still feel deep sadness, but the ability to perform this mental switch has made the process so much easier to bear.

Focus on what you've gained, not what you've lost.

KNOW YOU ARE STILL WORTHY

In Western culture, we tend to define ourselves by our occupation and position in society. It's no wonder, then, that a diagnosis of illness and disability or a life blow-up can completely shake your confidence and sense of self. It can be helpful to draw a line between your old life and your new life. Try not to compare your life now with what it was in the past, what you thought it would be or what your friends are doing (social media can make this particularly tricky). I call this mode of thought 'compare and despair'. Yes, you are different now, but it's important to never think of yourself as less than what you had been before. What has been taken from one aspect of your life has been gained in others. You will notice life becoming less about achieving status and accumulating things and more about appreciating and giving. We learn to find joy in simply being. Through our struggles we cultivate deeper, more enduring qualities that can never be taken away. Compassion, resilience, patience and humour have strength beyond measure and are the very marrow of being human. You are not broken. You are enough, exactly as you are.

YOU DON'T HAVE TO BE HEALTHY TO BE HAPPY

One of the biggest lessons I ever learned was that happiness and health are not the same thing. I shifted my mindset from 'I'll be happy when I am well' to 'I can be happy in this very moment, despite the challenges I face'. This works not just for illnesses, but for all kinds of life crises. If we future-date our happiness to a time that is dependent on something out of our control, we will always suffer. Don't decide you'll be happy when … 'I lose weight'; 'the global pandemic is over'; 'my partner stops doing this'. Instead, choose to be perfectly happy with your imperfect life. Start right now.

SET ACHIEVABLE GOALS DAILY

Your life has changed. Maybe a lot, maybe a little. To save a lot of pain and anguish, it's important to recalibrate your goals and expectations to suit these new circumstances. I suggest setting two or three small goals each morning. Write your daily goals down in a dedicated notebook in the morning and cross them off each evening. Depending on your individual circumstances, it could be things like taking the dog for a short walk, catching up with a friend, working on a creative project, or doing 15 minutes of gentle yoga. Choose goals that are realistic for your current situation and that will give you an internal boost. Even though you may have limited energy, if you are able to direct it into things that make your life richer or encourage you to grow as a person, then it is a day well lived.

LET FEELINGS FLOW AND THEN LET THEM GO

Don't give your thoughts too much weight: let them come and go with minimal resistance. Try to see them for what they are – fleeting and somewhat random figments of the imagination. It may help to view your thoughts and emotions like weather patterns of the mind. One minute you may be having a blue-sky day and the next you could find yourself in the middle of a downpour. That's all perfectly normal and the nature of being human. The important thing is not to focus on the thoughts themselves, but how you respond to this ever-changing forecast. Unhook from the temptation to put on your raincoat and go trudging into the storm at the first sign of rain. Instead, just watch the clouds arise and disappear with curiosity, humour and grace. Just be chill with whatever comes up and don't take it too personally. Whether joy or sorrow, each feeling is beautiful in its own way and has something to teach us.

You don't have to be healthy to be happy.

CHANNEL YOUR INNER RUBBER DUCKY

A rubber duck is a Zen master in disguise. No matter what happens in its world, it will continue to bob about on the surface. The water may become treacherous and unpredictable; our duck may encounter waves and whirlpools that pull it off course, rock its balance or even drag it under. But eventually, our heroic little duck will pop back up and continue on its way. The rubber duck shows us that although we may encounter fearful and unpleasant situations, the best way through is not by resistance, but simply by accepting and floating.

Here's how to channel your inner rubber duck

STEP 1: Stop.

STEP 2: Take a deep breath in and out, letting your shoulders fall away from your ears with the exhale.

STEP 3: Say (either to yourself or out loud): 'I accept that I am feeling (insert word here), but instead of fighting it I'm going to accept and float through it.'

STEP 4: Visualise our rubber ducky friend or, if this doesn't work, picture yourself gently floating on smooth water.

STEP 5: Be confident in the knowledge that this uncomfortable feeling/thought is temporary and WILL pass.

EMBRACE THE JOMO

The opposite of FOMO (the Fear of Missing Out), JOMO (the Joy of Missing Out) is an acquired skill that has lifelong benefits. It is the intentional and heartening choice of saying no to things that are too draining or do not match up with your core values. The key is to own your decisions. Be all in. You don't need to be concerned with any other options. Don't spend any time looking for greener grass or entertaining thoughts of 'what if'. Instead, fully embrace what you are doing and revel in the joy of what is right in front of you.

PRACTISE KINDNESS

I've had these words, based on the teachings of Mother Teresa, pinned above my door for years:

> Spread love everywhere you go.
> First of all in your own house. Give love to your children,
> to your wife or husband, to a next-door neighbour.
> Let no one ever come to you without leaving better
> and happier. Be the living expression of kindness:
> kindness in your face, kindness in your eyes, kindness
> in your smile, kindness in your warm greeting.

It's a reminder that just because we are struggling, it doesn't mean we can't contribute in a positive way to the lives of those around us. I believe that being ill or going through a crisis can actually make us better friends/sisters/partners because we are not distracted by much of the day-to-day stuff that seems to fill our lives when we're on autopilot. We are able to slow down and really listen to what others are saying. Being fully present and practising active listening is often the very best gift you can give a loved one.

JUST ADD NATURE

The healing power of nature is profound and often overlooked. It all started with a study in 1984 that showed that surgery patients recovered quicker when their hospital room had a view of nature, compared with looking out at a brick wall. Since then, advances in neuroscience and psychology have spurred further research showing that time spent in nature can decrease stress hormones and mental fatigue, help lower blood pressure and heart rate, improve mood, and decrease recovery times for illness and injuries, along with many more benefits.

And before you say, 'But I live in the city. What about me?' I have some good news: these benefits can apply to urban settings too. Even if it's just standing barefoot on a patch of grass, feeling the sun warm your skin or watching clouds move across the sky, any time spent interacting with nature is a thumbs-up for your health.

As I was writing this chapter at our home in the rainforest, a family of cassowaries serendipitously appeared. I was completely overwhelmed with awe and gratitude for this amazing encounter, and it reinforced what I already knew – that nature is a tonic for the soul. It's like the reset button for the body and mind. It encourages you to engage with all of your senses and be fully present in the moment. To me, time with nature is a necessity not a luxury, and I prioritise it accordingly.

Nature is a tonic for the soul. It's like a reset button.

TIPS FOR CONNECTING WITH NATURE

> GO OUTSIDE AT EVERY OPPORTUNITY.

> LET NATURAL LIGHT IN.

> HAVE PLANTS IN THE HOUSE.

> HANG PICTURES OF NATURAL SCENES ON YOUR WALLS.

> LISTEN TO RECORDINGS OF NATURAL SOUNDSCAPES (OCEAN, RIVER, FOREST, AND SO ON).

> SIT OR LIE SO THAT YOU CAN SEE OUT OF A WINDOW AND INTO THE OUTSIDE WORLD.

> JOIN A COMMUNITY GARDENING OR TREE-PLANTING GROUP AND GET YOUR HANDS DIRTY.

> SPEND TIME WITH ANIMALS: LOOKING INTO YOUR DOG'S EYES ACTUALLY INCREASES YOUR FEEL-GOOD HORMONES. ★

WHEN THERE IS NO CLEAR ENDING

Sometimes the future is so loaded with uncertainty and fear that it seems there is no clear path forward. I struggled with and fought against my condition for a long time before I finally came to accept that this was to be my new 'normal'. I slowly realised that no amount of positive thinking, denial, sheer will or wishing it away could change my circumstances. Eventually I started to let go of my old expectations and priorities, which cleared the way for new, more helpful ways of being. I released the drive to return to my previous life and began to forge a new path: one centred around inner values and acceptance. This change in mindset rekindled a sense of personal agency that had been lost to me for a long time. It has allowed me to find joy and meaning despite my limitations. And I know you will too.

HOW YOUR FRIENDS CAN BE KICK-ARSE SUPPORT PEOPLE

Helping someone who is having a rough time can be hard. So let's talk about how the people around you can be the best support crew possible.

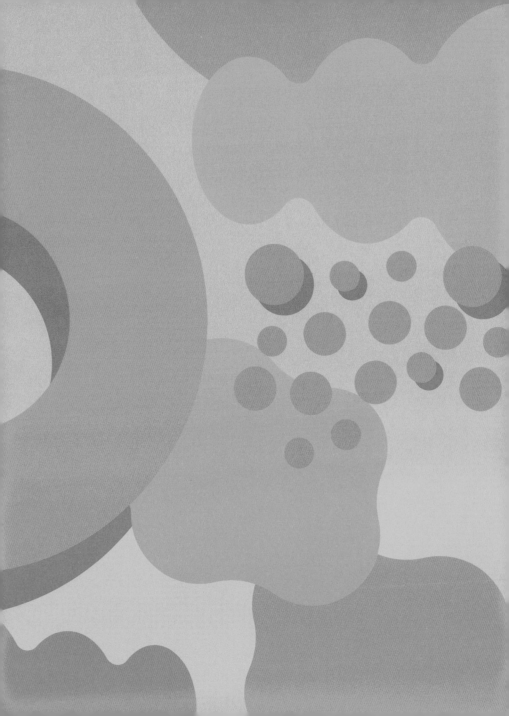

This section is for your friends and family. Perhaps ask them to have a read, or subtly leave it open on the kitchen bench with a giant sign beside it saying, 'Very important things to help me right now that I wish everyone around me knew'.

Love letter to my friends and family

Hello lovely support person

Here are a few thoughts and ideas to help you be a great support to someone you love who is going through a really sticky spot.

Look, it's really tough to get it right when you're supporting someone through a crisis; everyone is different and will want different things from you.

Know that you may not get it right and that's okay. As long as you are thoughtful and your intentions are good you just have to try your best with what you know.

Here are some things to keep in mind, some pitfalls to avoid and some super-awesome lovely ideas for things you can do to support.

Put a ring on it

Here's some truly awesome advice on the best way to have a big old whinge when life gets a bit squidgy. Created by clinical psychologist Susan Silk and mediator and author Barry Goldman, the 'Ring Theory' applies in any kind of crisis, and it's a great rule of thumb for helping to support someone in a crisis.

Here's how it works: the person who is going through the crisis is bang in the centre – they are the star of this shitshow. The ring around them represents their immediate family, partner and closest humans; their A-team. The next ring represents their friends, colleagues, etc.; the next-closest people.

Then the next ring – you get the idea – is people like Karen from Pilates and the handsome barista Ted. There is just one rule: comfort IN and dump OUT.

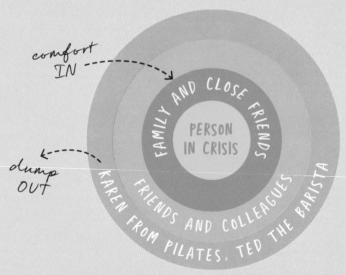

comfort
IN

dump
OUT

FAMILY AND CLOSE FRIENDS

PERSON
IN CRISIS

FRIENDS AND COLLEAGUES

KAREN FROM PILATES, TED THE BARISTA

Person in crisis

So the person at the centre of the crisis is allowed to whinge, moan and cry to anyone, in any ring. After all, they are the one in crisis and there's got to be some benefit to going through all this crap, right?

Everyone else

As for everyone else, well, they are also allowed to whinge, moan and cry to anyone, as long as that person is in a ring that is bigger than theirs.

For example, if you're really scared that a friend with a terrible illness might die, you should definitely not tell them that, it never goes down well. Don't mention it to their mum or brother or best mate, either; however, you could share your fears with your hairdresser or a loose acquaintance of the person in crisis, or even your own family. Someone in a bigger ring than you.

If you're talking to someone in a ring smaller than yours, then the goal is to listen and help. Not to give advice, or share your fears, but just to offer comfort.

Comfort in, *dump out.*

It's amazing how often people mix this up, which puts an unnecessary burden on the person in the centre of the crisis. So remember, before you speak, channel your inner Beyoncé and put a ring on it.

Sit in the rubble and acknowledge the pain

As humans we want to go straight into 'fix it' mode. We've been brought up in a culture where we are constantly told to 'look on the bright side' and cheer people up when they are down. That'll fix it. But sometimes the best way to help someone is to actually let them be in pain, because no matter what you say or do you can't take away their pain. It sounds counterintuitive, but it's actually much more helpful if you can instead acknowledge their pain and just let it exist.

Also, don't give advice.

This is true for just about every situation in life. Unless someone begs you for advice and really genuinely wants it, don't give it. You probably have a very insightful two cents' worth to throw into the mix, but unless you've done this exact thing before, your advice might not be very good anyway. And it could come back to bite you, if they follow your advice and it doesn't work for them. Often people have their own answers; they just need a chance to talk it out and articulate what they already know deep down. So listen, be interested. Ask questions.

A wise friend of mine, Tim, will always listen to what I have to say and, if he has something to add, he will offer, 'I've got some thoughts if you'd like to hear them?' Rather than pushing his ideas on me, he lets me decide whether or not I want to hear his thoughts and opt in.

My mum is, of course, excused from this rule because her advice is normally pretty bang on.

Here are some good questions you can ask:

What would you like to talk about?

How do you feel today?

What else would you like to talk about? Tell me more.

Would you like me to listen or offer some advice?

How to listen well

- Listen without judgement.
- Say less than the other person.
- Turn off devices.
- Repeat what they say, to acknowledge you have heard and understood.
- Keep your face neutral and friendly.*
- Be okay with silence.**

* You don't have to do a contorted upset face to show them you care. It can be distracting and feels inauthentic (and you'll get wrinkles in all the wrong places).

** Don't feel the need to frantically jump in to fill the spaces. From years spent interviewing people on camera, I've learned that often the most profound things are said in those silent spaces, when people just have a quiet reflective moment to let themselves think.

Don't try to fix me.

Just sit in the rubble with me, listen and hold my hand.

Say something

It can be really hard to know what to say when someone is going through an incredibly challenging time. Perhaps you think you'll upset them if you say something.

There are very few people in the world who, when faced with a challenging time, wouldn't want to know that people are thinking of them and sending them love. If you ignore it all together and don't acknowledge what has happened, it can feel really hurtful and dismissive. People who have lost a loved one often talk about the hurt they feel when they see friends or acquaintances who don't acknowledge their loss and avoid the conversation. It may be out of awkwardness, or not knowing what to say or worrying you'll upset them. But for the grieving person, not saying something is often worse.

For me, there were only a few people who, when I saw them after a long time, didn't acknowledge what I'd been through. It does hurt: it feels uncaring and dismissive. But even if you didn't do or say anything at the time and you're now feeling awkward, it's never too late to just say, 'I'm so sorry for what you had to go through.' Address the elephant in the room.

Maybe you feel like you don't know them well enough, or it's not your place. For me, though, it was actually the kindness that came from the most random places that was just as touching and sometimes even more so!

My dear friend Natasha was a rock to me throughout chemo. One day she bought me a gift with a card from one of her girlfriends, Roxy, whom I had never even met. The card read, 'I just wanted you to know that even people who don't know you are thinking of you and cheering for you and sending you love.' I was so incredibly touched.

If you're texting or emailing someone who is going through a tough time, remember not to burden the person by asking them something that requires a response, as that can create additional stress. So, unless it's appropriate, don't ask questions that warrant an immediate reply, such as, 'How are you?', 'What can I do to help?' or 'What's going to happen next?'. But you could say:

I'm so sorry you have to go through this.

No need to respond; I just want you to know that I love you and I'm thinking of you.

Just so you know, you're the bestest and it's just SOOO unfair you have to go through this.

I will love you every step of the way! You giant legend: you're going to smash this.

We haven't been in touch for a long time, but I heard the news and I want you to know that I am thinking of you and cheering for you and sending you love.

I cannot imagine what you are going through, but I want you to know you are so loved.

But avoid saying any of these things

Upsetting someone who is going through a major life crisis isn't going to win you a friendship bracelet (or feel particularly nice). So I'd strongly advise that you steer clear of any of these clichés.

Don't tell them, 'All things happen for a reason'.
Do they? Did I get cancer for a reason? Do people have horrific car accidents for a reason? It's something people say to fill the space, but it's supremely unhelpful and can sound dismissive of the immense pain someone might be experiencing. While good can eventually come from terrible times, there is no reason for this crisis. Put the phrase down and slowly back away.

Don't say, 'They only send it to the strong ones'.
Groan ... There is no one sitting up there saying, 'Oh, she's a tough cookie: let's give her cancer.' 'You know what, I reckon Brian could take it, let's give him a dose of bankruptcy and throw a marriage breakdown into the mix.' I mean, how unfair would that be? So just avoid it.

Don't try to fix it.
Because you can't. Nothing you say will fix it, so don't offer solutions, just listen and empathise.

Don't make it about yourself.
Don't tell them about the time you had a similar experience. Right now it ain't about you, so don't steal the spotlight – just listen and support.

'Your cancer diagnosis reminds me of the time I broke my arm ... I can really relate.'

Don't share a tragic story of your own (or someone else's).

Don't tell them about someone you know who died of the same thing or had an awful time (unless there is a kick-arse ending about how they beat it, met the love of their life – a handsome prince from a small country we've never heard of – had adorable twins and was given a small island).

Don't tell them to 'be positive'.

They are probably trying their best to do that already, so it's condescending. Also they may want to punch you in the face.

Don't tell them it will all be okay.

You may really believe this to be true or really want it to be true, but you don't know that. So it can come across as being dismissive and insincere, and they will lose trust in what you say.

Don't betray their confidence.

If they're sharing their vulnerabilities and fears, keep tight lips. Ask yourself if sharing the details would help the person or make them feel more anxious and upset?

In the case of illness, don't tell them about some magical cure you read about on the internet.

Unless you're their doctor, it's best to steer clear of any medical advice. Just leave it to them and their medical team.

Don't mention anything about it being 'God's plan'.

If you have a strong religious belief, that's great, but respect that the other person may not. They might also be a bit angry at God right now. One of my favourite cards, created by lymphoma survivor Emily McDowell of emandfriends.com, says: '*If this is God's plan, God is a terrible planner. (No offence if you're reading this, God. You did a really good job with other stuff, like waterfalls and pandas.)*'

And definitely don't say 'I'll do anything'

Instead, just DO something! While you might really mean it when you say, 'I'll do anything, just ask,' it puts the burden on the person going through the crisis to think of something and then ask you for it. Even during the toughest times, I didn't want to ring a friend and say, 'Would you mind bringing me dinner tonight?' How awkward! But when a friend just dropped off dinner for me, it was the greatest thing ever. If you're unsure if the person would be okay with it, offer something specific but give them an option. You've instantly taken the burden off them; they still might say no, but you've tried!

Here are some real-life things you could offer:

I'm at the supermarket; do you need me to grab you anything?

Need me to bring you anything from work?

Can I come over and water your plants?

Hey, I was planning on dropping you around some dinner tonight: would you prefer lasagne or salad?

Hey, I was going to pop past with some treats: fruit or chocolate?

Any appointments I can drive you to this week?

I have some time so I could pop over and help with your household chores: need the garden done, or the laundry?

Some other ideas you can steal from my family and friends:

Practical makes perfect

- Create them some custom playlists: one for strength, one for chilling, one for releasing, one for joy.

- Offer to come to an appointment and be a scribe.

- We all have to eat three times a day. Home-made meals (or fun snacks) dropped off are always awesome.

- Be a life-admin fairy. Sort out their gym membership, cancel some subscriptions, or ask if there are any other adminy-type things that need to be done.

- Send them a voice message or video message of support.

- Text them links to podcasts or funny videos.

- Make a folder of all their paperwork and a paper and digital calendar for their appointments.

- Be in contact frequently: use cards, letters, texts, frequent checking in. It helps so much!

- Offer to personally chauffeur them to important appointments or events. (You could even arrive with their name written on a sign, for a laugh. One of my excellent friends did this.)

Everyone loves a gift (unless you're Marie Kondo)

You can never go wrong with flowers or a small plant – they always brighten a day. Here are some other great gift ideas:

- Something bright, colourful and happy for their room
- If they're ill, a nice comfy chair for their bedroom so visitors can sit with them
- Personalised care packages – I LOVED getting these (make-up packs, stacks of magazines, a book, handwritten quotes)
- Massage or spa vouchers
- A spontaneous trip to get mani–pedis
- A subscription for audiobooks or to a music- or video-streaming service
- Movie vouchers
- Organise a library card for them – most libraries now have apps so you can borrow audiobooks and ebooks, and even read magazines and newspapers online. Libraries rock!
- A book of beautiful quotes
- A meaningful piece of jewellery, such as from thegivingkeys.com, where profits help others in need
- A stunning scarf from braveryco.com.au
- A crafty kit so they can get busy with their hands
- A book pillow (yeah, it's a thing, it holds your book up so you don't have to)
- Supersoft PJs and a robe to rest in, if they might be spending a bit of time in them … dreamy!

If you're buying for someone with cancer, make sure it's nothing strongly scented as everything smells pongy when you are going through chemotherapy.

Set up a network of love

Life gets busy and there's only so much you can do on your own to support someone else. Try setting up a 'network of love' to coordinate everyone who wants to do something. Create a calendar so there is always someone to spend time with the person, drop off meals or check in on them.

The network could last for a few months or much longer. It helps spread the load and allows people to be involved if they want to contribute but don't know what to do. Even if it's as simple as sending the person a text or phoning each day, having a plan is helpful and will make that person feel so supported.

My amazing friend Natasha arranged for all my friends to give me camera equipment so I could film my experience. It was awesome! Also, my boyfriend at the time, Roger, coordinated my friends to do something together for each round of chemo. It was incredibly creative and thoughtful, and gave me a huge boost each time. The network effect was powerful and made me feel so supported and loved. Here's what they did:

> ALL MY FRIENDS MADE ME A FUNNY VIDEO WITH MESSAGES OF SUPPORT.

> THEY CREATED A PLAYLIST OF SONGS AND EACH PICKED A SONG WITH A MESSAGE OR MEANING.

> MY FRIENDS, SQUASH BUDDIES AND WORK COLLEAGUES WENT TOGETHER TO DONATE BLOOD.

> THEY SPELLED OUT 'WE LOVE YOU' WITH THEIR BODIES IN A SERIES OF PHOTOS.

The muffin effect

My mum reckons you can connect with just about anyone with a tray of muffins, and I reckon she's right. When we were young, she used to bake muffins and take them wherever we were going: to the doctor, the dentist, our teachers. During my treatment the muffins evolved to date and cacao balls (you know, the hipster ones you see in cafés for $4 a pop). Every time we went to the hospital or an appointment, Mum would whip up a batch of these fancy-shmancy bliss balls.

She'd make a big jarful and give them to the nurses, doctors and hospital staff and sometimes even my fellow patients and their families. They were a hit! Every time we came into the hospital we'd be greeted by an eager sea of smiles; that's Mum, sprinkling kindness and thoughtfulness wherever she goes. There she was, coping with so much as a parent with a child going through chemo and treatment, and yet her thoughts were on helping the people who were helping us.

I was pretty shocked to hear from some of the nurses how poorly they are often treated by patients and their families. Not that they complained, but I asked them about it. One nurse mentioned that it's sometimes as though people mistake the 'H' in hospital for a hotel, treating the nurses more like resort staff.

Look, I understand that most people hanging out in a hospital are not having the greatest time of their lives, but my mind boggles at how people could ever treat nurses and doctors poorly. They are really angels on Earth. It was a great lesson I learned from my mum, to be serving and thinking of others even in your most challenging times. And it made the whole experience much more fun!

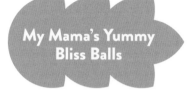

My Mama's Yummy Bliss Balls

INGREDIENTS

1 cup (160 g) Medjool dates

1 cup (100 g) almond meal

½ cup (35 g) shredded coconut, plus extra to roll the finished balls in

⅓ cup (35 g) rolled oats

⅓ cup (80 ml) coconut oil

⅓ cup (40 g) cacao powder

Optional extras: at your whim, feel free to add a tablespoon of chia seeds, protein powder, or psyllium for extra fibre.

1 Soak the dates in a small amount of warm water for about an hour. Drain excess water (and remove seeds if they happen to have them).

2 Blend up the dates, almond meal, coconut, oats, coconut oil and cacao until the mixture becomes sticky.

3 Put some shredded coconut into a small bowl.

4 Wet your hands so the mixture doesn't stick to them. Roll tablespoonfuls of mixture into balls with your hands, then roll them in the extra shredded coconut. Store in an airtight container in the fridge for up to 5 days.

Delight everyone and feel like a domestic goddess/god.

Be there once the storm has blown over

There is often a rush to offer support and love at the start of a crisis, which is great. But so often, it's after the initial crisis, when everything has calmed down a bit, that the person still needs ongoing support.

I know that for me, the toughest time was when I finished chemotherapy – which was a surprise to me. I thought I was through the worst of it and that it was time to just snap back into life as 'normal'. But my life had been flipped upside down. Now I had time to process it and work out what on earth I was going to do next. I had moved back to my flat in Sydney, gone through a break-up, was living with people I didn't know, had really low energy and was trying to get back into part-time work and be motivated and do social activities and, well ... it was a LOT. That was the toughest time emotionally, and when I really needed support. I was really lonely and felt lost.

NINJA TIP

Set a reminder on your phone to check in on your friend every few days or weekly. You can forget, in the busyness of life, to connect and reach out, especially once the initial drama is over. Setting reminders for key milestones, events, appointments or just a regular check-in time is a great way to remind yourself to be a great support person.

Always be kinder than necessary

Three weeks into chemo, I still had long hair and, to the outside world, looked totally normal, even well. Meanwhile, I was being pumped full of toxic chemicals and drugs and felt like I had the worst hangover of my life, which would just NEVER go away. Oh, and that minor concern that I wasn't entirely sure I'd be alive by next Christmas. It was a great reminder that you never know what someone is going through. So it can never hurt to be a little kinder than necessary.

I saw when I went through chemo how much kindness does exist in the world. You see it in people's eyes – not pity, but a genuine desire to make your day easier. You can see people's humanity. Perhaps we just need to treat everyone, always, as though they are more precious and delicate than we realise. Default to love.

It's so easy to judge someone, but everyone is going through their own battles all the time. Relationship breakdowns, the loss of a spouse, mental health issues, overwhelm. Life can be tricky and hard at times, and it is often then that the smallest gestures of kindness can really make your day.

So be kind, it's rockstar!

You've been through a rough time.

But remember, it's not the whole book – it's just one chapter in your unfolding story.

THE NEXT AWESOME CHAPTER OF YOUR LIFE

After a major life upheaval, remember that there is no rush to have all the answers and know where everything will lead. These are some concepts that have helped me as I've learned to move at a more sustainable pace.

Feeling icky again

On the road to recovery I've crashed and burned more times than I can remember. Two years of pushing really hard to live my #bestlife post-chemo had left me feeling totally depleted and despairing. Would I ever feel good again?

I was waking up feeling nauseous most days and I had no energy whatsoever. I was struggling with serious fatigue, exacerbated by stress and overwhelm. I was feeling very flat, mentally, and was just finding it really hard to be motivated to do anything. Under the directions of a holistic doctor, I cut out dairy, wheat, alcohol, caffeine and sugar (all the fun things). Sure chemo was tough, but have you tried weaning yourself off coffee? My new doctor prescribed me three naps a day and a 9 pm bedtime (which was really hard for this night owl) as well as some supplements for my gut health, adrenal glands and fatigue.

Once more I was forced to prioritise my health to number one (how was it not already?) but even after what I've been through it is so easy to slip back into the dangerous habits of putting our health on the sideline as we get really 'busy and important'. I'd just started a new business creating high-quality videos for clients that involved intense production schedules; I wanted to deliver exceptional work. On top of that I was trying to be social and make new friends, get back on the dating scene, improve my squash (lol), mentor some up-and-coming creatives and do volunteer tutoring. I'd even begun training for a half marathon (what was I thinking?).

I'd exhausted myself all over again. It finally dawned on me that the business-as-usual approach to my life was not working and if I continued to live the way I always had, then there was a danger I could make myself really sick again. I've now had to accept that my life needs to move at a different pace; that I'm dealing with a form of chronic fatigue and I have to stop pushing against it and once more accept it and go with the flow.

NINJA TIP

Get into the habit of stopping, resting and recuperating before you feel sick and tired, not after.

Note to future self

Please never forget that self-care and good health has to take priority every day. Carve out space for meditation, exercise, stretching and resting each day.

Prioritise being organised to have nourishing food around. All of the other fun, shiny, exciting things you want to do just have to come after those primary (slightly boring, but very important) things.

You will be a better partner, friend, family member and citizen of the world when you are not in survival mode, but instead feel well, have energy and can face the day feeling strong and energised.

Got it? Good.

Write a love letter to your body

Promise to love, cherish and support your body, and give it what it needs. You're going to be so disappointed with yourself if, many years down the track, you end up sick and unwell and you could have done something now to prevent it. Exhausting your human capital for the sake of a job or relationship is just never worth it. It doesn't matter what has happened before now, where you're at or how far off course you feel you have come. You can start now. Your body and mind will love you for it.

A greater love, respect and care for my body has certainly been one of the biggest shifts to come out of this entire experience, for me. And I believe that building your physical and mental strength while the sun shines is one of the greatest acts of self-care and love you can do, so you are strong no matter the weather.

It's so easy to slip back into old habits but what do we really have if we give away our health?

Take a moment to sit down and write to your body; tell it what a rock star you think it is.

To my dear darling body,

I just wanted you to know how much
I appreciate, respect and love you.

Thank you for lungs that allow me to breathe,
talk to those I love and sing (really well,
according to my mum and not my sisters).

Thank you for a strong heart that beats
today and gives me the gift of life.

Thank you for strong legs that allow me to
move about this world and explore and adventure.

Thank you for everything you have gotten
me through. Thank you for healing and mending me
when I felt broken, for pulling me through and giving
me a second crack at life. I'm so grateful to be here.

I promise to stop being so harsh on you and
instead focus on all the things I love about you.

I promise to appreciate you, look after you,
nourish and protect you into the future.

I promise to love all the parts of you; for we are in this
together on our short and precious ride through life.

I feel grateful to have you, as you are, right now.

Lots of love from me
(which is also you, but ... you know).

You're awesome!
xxxxx

Your body is telling you things all the time.

But
are
you
listening?

Listening to your body

A wise person, when asked what most puzzled him about humans, responded, 'Man, because he sacrifices his health in order to make money; then he sacrifices money to recuperate his health.'

Mad, but so true! We run ourselves into the ground until we are achy and sore and tired. Then we throw money at the problem: going to doctors, specialists and physiotherapists; buying all kinds of drugs and painkillers that we need to try to recuperate. It's a bit loony when you put it like that, isn't it?

We're living in an era when so many of us are rushing at such a frantic pace that we don't have the time or space to check in and listen to our bodies. But what is actually more important than the health of our body?

What are you trying to tell me, dear body?

I have a much closer relationship with my body now than I ever had before. I'm better at tuning in to it and thinking about what it needs. When I get a headache or an aching shoulder I think of it as a small nudge or alert from my body. Instead of going straight to painkillers, numbing it and going out to that social engagement, I think, 'What is my body trying to tell me? That it needs more sleep? More water? Some quiet time out?' I try to listen to what it is telling me and then – here is the hard part – doing as it says.

Often it doesn't fit in with my social plans and I'm certainly not yet an angel in putting my body first and foremost. Sometimes it's not 100 per cent practical to do that. But health and energy have been promoted to the top of my list of things I give a damn about.

We all need to get better at listening to our bodies, like really listening. Not the kind of listening you do when you're on the phone to a friend but scrolling through Instagram. Actually listening and then, more importantly, doing as it asks!

A few ways to help you listen to your body

- Try daily meditation.
- Do some stretches or yoga in the morning to check in with how your body is feeling.
- Have scheduled times in your day when you stop and breathe and check in (if you're forgetful like me, set a reminder on your phone).
- When you eat, focus on just eating and put the phone away. Notice how you feel 30 minutes after eating. Start to get clear on what foods make you feel good and what foods don't agree with you.

How is your body feeling right now? What messages is it sending you? What feels good? What doesn't? What tweaks to your daily routine could help it feel better?

You are the world's leading expert on you

Congratulations! It turns out you're the expert on what it's like to live inside that body of yours. You're the only one who knows what's normal and what's not. Be polite to medical experts always, but be demanding. Keep digging and asking questions until you have answers. Many doctors are used to seeing the 'worried well', people who are healthy but think there is something wrong with them, so if you really know you are not well you have to speak up! You have to be your own advocate, because – as clever as doctors are – they are only going off the information you provide and their past experiences and knowledge.

If I had my time again, rather than passively listening to my doctors when they dismissed my early symptoms, I wish I had found the confidence to say:

This is having a severe impact on my life.

I really need a better solution here.

I'm in immense pain.

I'm sick all the time and I'm not getting any better.

What would you do if this was you?

I'm waking up every single night from the pain and drenching sweats.

What is the next step?

Before you go to a doctor or specialist, gather your thoughts. Write out all of your current symptoms and issues, and the questions you want to ask. How often do you leave the doctor's rooms and think, 'Damn, I forgot to ask about that weird pain in my toe ...'

Crank up the dramah!

Gals, we need to learn from our male friends and crank up the dramah a few notches when we're not feeling well.

You know what they can be like when they have Man Flu: 'I don't think anyone has ever suffered as I have, etc. etc.' In fact, one of the most popular videos I've ever made was about the dreaded Man Flu: 50 million views show that a lot of women can perhaps relate.

(No offence to the blokes reading this. I'm sure you're real tough and not at all like those other snowflakes.)

Be a teensy bit hypochondriac

I often joke to friends now that I don't think it hurts to
be just a little bit of a hypochondriac. Women in particular
should be a little less stoic and have a dash more drama about
their health.

Gabrielle Jackson, the author of *Pain and Prejudice*,
explains that 'women wait longer for pain medication than
men, wait longer to be diagnosed with cancer, are more likely to
have their physical symptoms ascribed to mental health issues'.
On top of all that, she describes that many women are living in
constant pain and are not even aware that it isn't normal. (Wow,
that reminds me of someone!) An editorial published in the *New
England Journal of Medicine* even revealed that women are
seven times more likely than men to be misdiagnosed and
discharged during an ACTUAL HEART ATTACK!!! Holy hell, that's
serious. So for the ladies reading, you HAVE to find your voice:
it's literally a matter of life and death.

Many of the chronic pain conditions that affect women –
endometriosis, fibromyalgia and chronic fatigue syndrome,
to name a few – have similar symptoms, and if you have one
you are also more likely to be affected by others.

*You are your own best advocate,
so speak up and keep asking questions.*

If you are feeling unwell over an extended period of time and you cannot get to the bottom of it:

- Make sure you find a doctor you really 'click' with, who takes your pain or issue seriously. (If need be, get a second, third or 197th opinion.)

- Become the world's best note-taker, so you have really clear information on your symptoms, your diet, your sleep and any other strange and unusual things that are going on. (Keep notes on your phone or in a notepad.)

- Even better, grab your phone and film yourself explaining exactly how you're feeling as the symptoms arise. (When you are crook it can all become a hazy blur and, if a picture paints a thousand words, I reckon a video paints a million.)

- Go and see a vet. (Just kidding, but it was my vet dad and my persistent mother who did get me diagnosed in the end. The point being, keep digging and getting other opinions.)

Do not wear make-up to the doctor. Yeah, that bronzer makes you look like a glowing beach babe, but it also makes you look a million bucks when you actually feel like a squashed cucumber, and it can give your doctor a bum steer. So don't let it work its magic and bewilder your doctor when you're trying to get to the bottom of what is going on. Let your pasty, lovely, exhausted face do the talking.

Treat your body like a Ferrari

I'm no car connoisseur, but if you were given a car at 18 and told it was the only one you would have for life, you'd take pretty damn good care of it. You'd put only the best fuel in it and you wouldn't let its tank run low. You'd do consistent maintenance and make sure it had everything it needed to run smoothly. I mean, you're going to be still driving this car at 80 or if you're lucky into your nineties. Your body is the only one you get and yet often you're more likely to be doing burnouts on an empty tank of crappy fuel than giving it what it needs.

As with so many other things in Western culture, we are usually waiting for a total breakdown before we act! Instead we need to be going to the mechanic for constant maintenance, rather than waiting for the engine to blow up.

Make sure you're giving your machine what it needs to hum along beautifully.

Is your engine firing on all cylinders right now? What could you change to look after yourself better?

Don't wait for a
total breakdown
before you act.

Human Body User Manual
FOR OPTIMAL PERFORMANCE

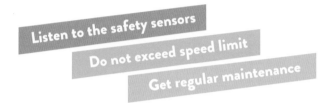

Keep it moving

Love it or hate it, you've just got to do it. If you are physically able, exercise is not just an option, it's a compulsory insurance policy for the future and something you owe to your body. Rejoice that you have the ability and opportunity to do this. Not everyone is so lucky! It's estimated that about a third of cancers can be prevented through exercise and a healthy diet and, trust me, if you can avoid the big C you really wanna do that! The Cancer Council recommends a minimum 30 minutes of moderate exercise every day, or 60 minutes to reduce your risk of cancer. So find something you love. You might hate running; that's fine, you don't have to do it! Maybe you need a group sport or a gym class or yoga, Prancercise (google it) or TAPfit (it's a thing, check it) – find something you feel motivated to do, and do it.

Use only the best fuel

A good diet is essential to building up mental and physical resilience. We now know that many foods have a direct correlation to mental wellbeing.

Every single body is different, so it's important to find what feels right for you and start to notice when different foods make you feel blergh. Many foods can cause inflammation in the body, which makes you feel rotten.

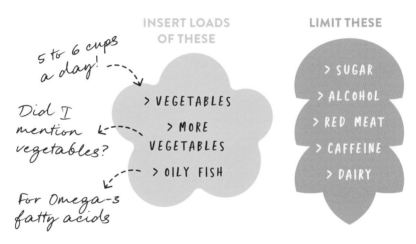

INSERT LOADS OF THESE

> VEGETABLES

> MORE VEGETABLES

> OILY FISH

LIMIT THESE

> SUGAR

> ALCOHOL

> RED MEAT

> CAFFEINE

> DAIRY

5 to 6 cups a day!

Did I mention vegetables?

For Omega-3 fatty acids

I'm not going to tell you to cut out meat altogether (you do you), but the Cancer Council advises limiting red-meat intake (such as beef, lamb and pork – they're classified as probable carcinogens, which means that excess consumption is linked to cancer). They recommend cutting out processed meats (bacon, ham, devon or fritz, kransky and frankfurts). The World Health Organization classes these as a group 1 carcinogen, which means that despite being totally delicious, there is evidence that they can also totally contribute to cancer.

Get enough H$_2$O in your system

It's so easy to forget to drink enough water each day. Make sure you always have a bottle with you when you leave the house, or if you work in an office have a bottle on your desk so you can keep the fluids going in. There are also great apps you can use to give you a little nudge to top up your H$_2$O.

Calm your engine

Oh, I know meditation can seem hard. Why is it, though, that every successful person seems to be into it? If you really can't wrap your head around meditation, find an activity that calms you: surfing, playing the guitar, sitting in nature or doing something with your hands. But make space each day to calm your mind.

Add 8 hours of rest

I know everyone bangs on about sleep and it's really boring and you think, 'I KNOW!' But if you're not getting your eight hours, then you are putting your engine at serious risk of disease. I'm so passionate about this that it's getting its own page, coming up.

Add additional stationary periods

It's actually okay to rest! Did you know that? I didn't allow myself to do this until recently. Naps are good for you. Neuroscience tells us that the optimal nap time is for less than 30 minutes and before 3 pm, so it doesn't affect your most important sleeping periods.

Remove stressors

I've been in toxic jobs that I know without a doubt have compounded my health issues. Can I just let you know now that NO JOB is worth jeopardising your health, no matter how much you love it. While you are in it you can't see the forest for the trees, but a toxic boss or workplace is rarely going to get better. Start looking for something else, and in the interim try not to take on the negativity of the situation, prioritise your health and get the hell out of there! The same goes for toxic relationships: they're lethal and compromise our immune system.

Disconnect the engine

Have a phone-free day (or at least half day) once a week. Have a turn-off point for your phone. If you're really struggling, you can make the screen greyscale. The average Australian spends a full day on their phone PER WEEK – that is OVER A MONTH OF YOUR YEAR! Imagine what you could do with that time. Learn a language? Write a book? Spend it with those you love?

Do not exceed the speed limit

Would you please just slow it allll downnn? This frantic rushing around is making us sick. It stimulates cortisol and keeps our bodies constantly drained. I try to channel this advice from St Francis de Sales whenever I can:

> DO NOT BE IN A HURRY; PEACE, CALM, AND REST
> OF MIND ARE PRECIOUS, AND THE TIME YOU SPEND
> IN QUIETNESS WILL BE TIME WELL SPENT.

If you're not where you'd like to be today, DO NOT FRET! Make a promise to yourself to look after your greatest gift, begin tinkering with your engine and making improvements. Start small, but start now. Your health needs to be your number-one priority, if you plan on giving yourself the best shot at living a long, happy, pain-free life.

Charge your batteries first

When your phone is about to die and is on 2 per cent battery, I'm sure you'll agree it's not the time to lend someone else your charger. If they're like most people they'll forget to give it back and then you will die – well, your phone will die. Okay, a tad dramatic, but you catch my drift. Your energy is such a precious commodity that you really shouldn't be giving it to anyone else unless you are fully charged. (For parents, of course you have adorabubble little dependants to factor into this mix. But you deserve the time and space to recharge where possible too.)

Once you have your energy topped up and you have an overflow, that's when you can share it with your most important humans. When they're all charged up, you can give it to your next nearest and dearest people and only if there is anything left over should it go to other people. Don't do the 'jerk' manoeuvre of giving your best energy to people who are loose acquaintances and then treating your besties poorly. So easy to do but it's all the wrong way around!

So what charges your batteries? And what drains them?

Getting clear on what drains you and what energises you is the first step to taking control of your energy. In order to do that, however, there is a two-letter word you need to become more familiar with (turn to page 162).

> Write down ten of your favourite things in the world to do. What would the perfect day of recharging look like for you?

WHAT CHARGES YOU UP?

> EXERCISE

> STRETCHING AND YOGA

> SOULFUL CONVERSATIONS
  WITH BEST FRIENDS

> BEING IN NATURE

> LEARNING AND GROWING

> READING

> PLAYING WITH
  AN ADORABLE DOG

> LISTENING TO A PODCAST

> MAKING A RIDICULOUSLY
  SILLY TIKTOK WITH
  YOUR SISTER! (JUST ME?)

> BEACH AND SUNSHINE

WHAT DRAINS YOU?

> GOSSIPING

> HANGING OUT WITH
  NEGATIVE PEOPLE

> DRINKING TOO MUCH

> EATING JUNK FOOD

> ATTENDING STRESSFUL EVENTS

> READING TOO MUCH
  NEGATIVE NEWS

> MINDLESSLY SCROLLING
  SOCIAL MEDIA

> WORKING LONG HOURS

> BAD DESK SET-UP THAT
  MAKES EVERYTHING ACHE

> BEING STILL FOR TOO LONG

That word that starts with N and ends with O

An illness gives you this new-found ability to say no to things you don't want to do. No one is going to argue with the chick who had cancer recently that they absolutely have to attend a birthday party/barbecue/wedding/new puppy shower (yeah, that's a thing). Ah, silver linings. But remember that permission slip we wrote ourselves at the start of the book? You've still got it.

What we say no to is just as important as what we say yes to. This includes relationships and friendships as well as commitments and events. Remember, you don't actually owe anyone anything. I massively struggled with this at first because I suffer terribly from FOMO and I do like to help others and contribute. I've learned, however, that if I spend all my time focused on others' needs, it doesn't leave me with the energy I need to do the things I'm really passionate about, and then I feel flat and drained and I'm really no good to anyone else anyway.

A girlfriend gave me a great analogy recently. She said, 'You have to put a value on your time. Imagine that an hour is worth $1000. Therefore, before you say yes to something, you can think, "Is this worth $1000 of my time?" If you don't value your time, no one will.'

You know when you were a kid and you'd just flat-out chuck a tantrum if you didn't want to do something? In case you forgot how to say NO the way you did when you were a sassy little kid, opposite are a few starters that don't involve spitting the dummy.

There is no hope in hell I'll be coming, but I still want to be invited.

WAYS TO SAY NO:

> NO THANKS.

> NOPE.

> I CAN'T, BUT THANKS!

> THANK YOU, BUT WORK AND FAMILY COMMITMENTS PREVENT ME AT THIS TIME.

> THANKS FOR THINKING OF ME, BUT I CAN'T AT THIS TIME.

> THANKS SO MUCH FOR THINKING OF ME, DARLING, BUT I'D RATHER POKE MY EYE OUT WITH A FORK. (OKAY, MAYBE DON'T USE THAT UNLESS YOU NEVER WANT TO BE INVITED AGAIN.)

Remember, you don't need to give a reason and you don't need to explain it away with a complex excuse for why you can't do it. If you don't want to, just say no. And if your body says NO then it is a no.

How often do you say yes to something and you can almost hear a deep internal groan, as though your body is saying, 'Do we havvveee to?' Well, you know what: no! You don't have to. (Unless you're in danger of becoming a total hermit and need to force yourself to have some human interaction.)

Take time to think about things if you don't need to give an immediate answer, but if you're quite sure it's a no, it's good to get back to people as quickly as you can.

When was the last time you said yes when you meant NO! What do you need to say no to in future?

Sleep your way to the top

Sleep really is my new best friend. A friend I'd neglected for most of my adult life, as I've always been a night owl. And if I'm totally honest, my phone addiction had made it far worse. There are so many distractions now that can steal our sleep from us. Netflix recently announced that its biggest competitor is sleep. Yikes! I'd always known that sleep and rest were important, but in my attempt to cram as much as possible into my days I thought, 'Well, what does it matter if I lose an hour here or there.' Well, it turns out it matters a huge amount.

For me, it was reading the book *Why We Sleep* by neuroscientist Matthew Walker that really changed my approach to sleep. According to Walker, routinely sleeping less than six or seven hours a night demolishes your immune system, doubles your risk of cancer and is a key determinant of whether or not you will develop Alzheimer's disease. Even a week of bad sleep disrupts blood-sugar levels so profoundly that you could be classified as prediabetic. Poor sleep also increases the risk that your coronary arteries will become blocked and brittle, setting you on a path towards cardiovascular disease, stroke and congestive heart failure, and it also contributes to major psychiatric conditions including depression and anxiety. Fun, fun, fun!

The thing that really took my breath away was understanding sleep's role in combating cancer. At night your body basically deploys these cancer-killing 007-style agents to go around and clear out the build-up of cancer-causing cells. If they don't get their full shift in, they simply can't get all the work done and so these dangerous nasty cells just build up. Like asking a cleaner to do an eight-hour job in four hours. They're not going to get into the corners or have time for dusting, and they won't have time to take the rubbish out. I thought about the years and years I'd underslept. I'm not saying it gave me cancer – we don't know what causes lymphoma – but I certainly never gave my body a chance to catch up by itself.

Sleep doesn't come easily to me, but so as to commit wholeheartedly to it I made it my word for an entire year. My one thing I would come back to and focus on. I'm still getting there and I'm far from the sleep guru I'd like to become, but here are some nuggets of sleep wisdom that have really helped me.

Sleep tips

- **Put your phone to bed at a set time in another room.**
- **Go to bed at the same time each night.**
- **Wear a night mask.**
- **During the week, say no to activities that will run too late, or just leave early.**
- **Wear earplugs (the gel ones that create a total vacuum in your ear). Bonus tip: wash them in soapy water each morning so they don't get nasty.**

Pick one thing this week that will help you get some more ZZZZs.

Feeling the Zen vibes

Here's how to think about meditating if you're having trouble 'getting it'. For busy go-getters, the idea of sitting down to do 'nothing' for 20 minutes can be almost anxiety-inducing. (I could be doing SO MUCH WITH THIS TIME, like kicking goals and working on plans – in reality you'd probably just waste 20 minutes scrolling Instagram.) It's hard if you are a must-erbator like me: you know, someone who feels like they 'must' do something every minute of the day.

But the benefits of meditation can be immense. I've learned the Vedic method of meditation. You meditate by repeating a mantra that your teacher gives you. The mantra is a vehicle that is meant to help get you started and take you to a place of inner contentment. Ideally, you do this for 20 minutes each morning and night.

There are many different types of meditation and ways to do it, as well as some great apps too!

Try to find a time each morning and night that you could commit to meditating. Start small, with just a few minutes, and build up.

If you're still not convinced or you struggle to get into meditation, here are a few thoughts I'm just going to leave here. My meditation teacher (and fellow lymphoma survivor) Mathieu taught me these things, as I try reallllyyy hard to become a meditator.

- Imagine a muddy glass of water: if you let it sit on the bench it becomes clear as all of the dirt settles to the bottom. That is what meditation does for your mind. It purifies your nervous system in order to help you to think clearly and therefore make better decisions for yourself.

- You don't like doing laundry, do you? (If you do, you need to get out more.) But you do like having nice clean clothes. It might feel a bit boring or hard, but the end result of having clean, nice-smelling clothing is what we want ... that is what meditation is like for your mind.

- Rather than think of it as doing 'nothing', think of it as giving a gift to your mind and body. Something that you owe to yourself. By doing 'nothing' we are doing so much. Giving our mind and body a chance to release all the stress that builds up. It's actually an act of wonderful self-care.

With a calm mind and body, you can take on the world.

That's enough todaying for today

In a world where we are connected 24/7, creating your own boundaries is so important for good emotional, mental and physical health. Having a clear cut-off point for your day is key. Especially for entrepreneurs, creatives, business owners or any human with a job or family ... yeah, everyone. Remember that when you die, your Inbox is still going to be full; there is literally a never-ending list of things you could do each day. To live well and sustainably you need to give your brain a vacay each night.

WAYS TO SWITCH OFF FROM THE DAY

> WRITE A TA-DA LIST OF EVERYTHING YOU GOT DONE TODAY.

> WRITE A LIST OF EVERYTHING THAT CAN WAIT UNTIL TOMORROW.

> HAVE A CLEAR END POINT TO YOUR WORK DAY. MAYBE THAT IS GOING TO THE GYM AFTER WORK, OR IF YOU WALK HOME, IT MIGHT BE A STATUE YOU PASS THAT MEANS THE WORK DAY IS OVER.

> CHANGE YOUR CLOTHES (ESPECIALLY IF WORKING FROM HOME).

> HAVE A BEDTIME FOR YOUR PHONE WHEN IT GETS TURNED OFF AND LEFT SOMEWHERE OTHER THAN YOUR BEDROOM TO CHARGE. EVEN THE PRESENCE OF A PHONE IS TAKING AWAY YOUR BRAIN ACTIVITY AND ABILITY TO CONNECT.

Daily rituals to make you feel great

I'm certainly not saying I nail each of these every day, but when I've got these under control and do them daily, I feel calm, in control and have a more joyful day.

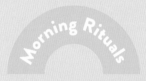

- **Drink a glass of warm water.**
- **Do a body scan to see how you're feeling. Feel grateful for what feels good.**
- **Smile to yourself and give thanks for the gift of this day (even a fake smile helps).**
- **Meditate for 20 minutes.**
- **Make the bed (look at you kicking goals already).**
- **Do morning stretches or yoga.**
- **Journal or write morning pages for 20 minutes.**
- **Have a nutritious breakfast.**
- **Listen to some upbeat tunes and have a daggy dance party for one.**

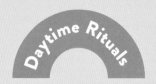

Daytime Rituals

Get some fresh air. Get out of your workplace and get some fresh air every day, no matter what! The time you spend out of the office will refresh your brain a million times over.

When you eat, just eat. Don't try to do three million other things; your brain and body deserve a small parcel of time to switch off and be present in the task of eating.

Move every hour. Set a reminder to stretch your neck and arms, do a lap around the office or have a spontaneous dance break. I once heard of an office that does a one-minute disco, complete with flashing lights and disco ball, at random times throughout the day. That's my kind of workplace!

Breathe. Set reminders to do some deep breathing. How often do you really properly breathe during the day?

Mindful moments. Find times to stop during the day and really take in the details of the moment you are in. What can you appreciate about your life and where you are right now?

Nap. Have a short 20-minute rest if your work set-up allows. (This could be in the park if you work in an office, or maybe you could campaign for a nap room.)

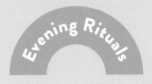

- Prepare lunch and healthy snacks for the next day.
- Get your clothes ready for the next day.
- Put your phone to bed by 8 pm (earlier if you can).
- Put a glass of water beside your bed for the morning.
- Put everything in your room back in its place (calm space, calm mind).
- Read for 30 minutes.
- Think of the things you're grateful for in your life and send out thoughts and wishes to the people you love.

This breathing technique, alternative nostril breathing, is great for an instant chill, and was taught to me by my yoga teacher, Kate Kendall.

Have a breather

Get into a comfortable position and exhale completely. Then cover up the right nostril with your right thumb and inhale through the left nostril.

Then cover your left nostril and exhale through the right nostril. Then send it back, so inhale through the right nostril, then cover the right nostril and exhale through the left nostril. That is one round.

I find even just doing it a few times is a great way to calm myself down at the end of the day.

THINKING ABOUT THE FUTURE

A few other things I'd really like to
say before we wrap this baby up.

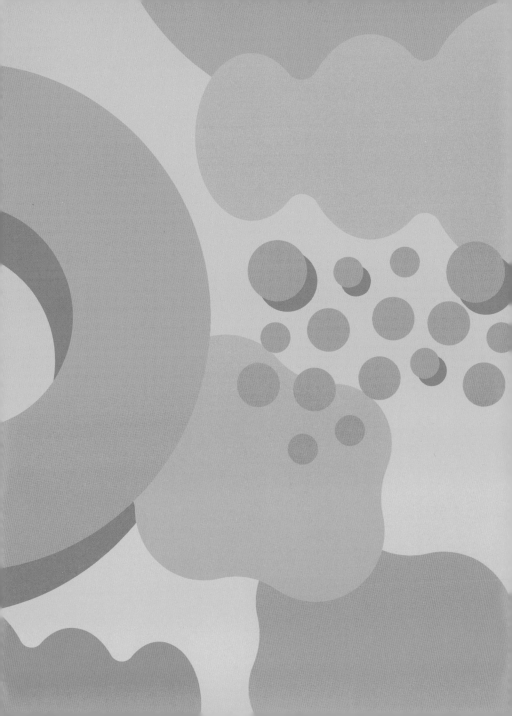

Be in control of your own destiny

If you've already had kids and don't want any more, or if you're not remotely interested in bringing more little anklebiters onto the planet, then feel free to ignore the following advice. But otherwise, whether you're a woman, or a man who would like to have a baby with a woman one day, read on.

Freezing my eggs was not something I had been thinking of doing at 31. But now I've done it, I'm so glad I had the opportunity; it's given me such comfort knowing I have them there as a backup option. But it got me thinking about how, as a young woman of 'child-bearing age', I was so uninformed about the whole process. With many women now pursuing careers they love and, for the first time in human history, pushing childbirth back, somewhere along the way we forgot to talk to young women and men about planning for a family, and realistic timeframes if they do indeed want to become a parent one day.

My gynaecologist Bill thinks that all women around the 30-year-old mark who plan on having children one day should get an Anti-Mullerian Hormone test (AMH test) to get a clearer picture of their options. In an eggshell, it's a simple blood test that can measure the number of eggs you have left. It's not foolproof and doesn't tell you about the quality of the eggs, but it can give you an insight into the remaining quantity of eggs and the number of fertile years you may have left. It's a good starting point to indicate if there might be any problems down the track, so you can be aware of what you're dealing with, rather than flying blind and crossing all your fingers and toes that you will find someone your parents would approve of, without face tattoos or a gambling debt, to procreate with in a timeframe that aligns with your fertility window.

Bill reckons getting healthy 30-year-olds to do any kind of future screening is tough because we all think we're invincible (I mean, never in a million years did I think I'd get cancer), but be a legend and buck the stereotype, would you, and get a clear picture of your options.

Do you want children? *If so ideally what age do you want to be having kids?*

Are you aware of your own fertility? *Would you like to know your options and timeframes?*

Would you consider having them without a partner? *You need to get clear on what you want.*

If you're not sure what to do, a good starting point might be to talk to your doctor or GP about what options are available.

I have a bunch of girlfriends who, since I got cancer, have investigated their own fertility options. For some it's been fine – they've got a good amount of eggs in reserve and have a good timeframe ahead of them before they need to start having a family – while others have gone through the egg-freezing procedure or even made embryos with their current partner. Another has decided to get donor sperm and start a family by herself straight away, as her fertility window was much smaller than she had realised. I just think, at the end of the day, if you plan on having kids it's good to be in charge of your options so you have the most choices possible! (It will also give you clarity about who you want to be with and perhaps prevent you wasting time with someone whose values and timeframe don't align with yours.)

I've heard some women express shame about the need to get their eggs frozen and I really think there is no need to feel that. You haven't failed at life because you aren't married and shacked up by 35 with three kids, a dog and a picket fence. You might not be ready for kids yet, or perhaps your career is at its peak and that's your priority right now. And it can be really hard to find the right person: the odd scroll through a dating app is enough to turn you off for life (really, Kevin, do you honestly think that photo with your tongue out giving the finger is going to be a hit with the ladies? You are 43 ... get it together, mate). Finding someone you want to create a mini-me with and possibly spend the rest of your life with isn't exactly a small decision. So remember that exploring your fertility choices is not shameful and there are no bad options, just different methods, so you're free to do what's best for you at the time.

If you're financially in the position to do so and you're keen to investigate further, you could instead think about it as an awesome backup plan, created by a clever, kick-arse woman who is keeping her options open.

Anyway, rant about fertility over: in summary, be in control of your own destiny! And hypothetical adorable future children.

> You might not be ready for kids, but do you think it could be helpful to explore your fertility options?

Do something that matters

No one is going to say at your funeral: 'She hit her sales targets every month and will be forever remembered for all the unpaid overtime and weekends she worked. What a human!'

Did you know she had a thigh gap all her life?

He made two million dollars a year.

Of all that you have done in your life so far, what are you most proud of? That's a great starting point to think about what is truly meaningful to you, what gives you purpose and what drives you. It might be being a brilliant and loving family member or being an amazing parent and raising beautiful children. Or growing a business that delivers a great service to many. Maybe it's about creating impact in your community.

I've always wanted to help make positive change in the world through the power of communication. I've worked with lots of amazing campaign organisations such as SumOfUs, GetUp, the Climate Council, World Wildlife Fund and other dynamic startups that are working to make positive change in the world.

When I think about what I'm most proud of in my life so far, it's being involved in creative video campaigns that have made an impact in the world. And the great relationships I've formed doing that work (as well as the joy and purpose I've experienced from mentoring and supporting others in their careers). This is something that I'm sure will keep evolving for me as I keep learning and growing.

What do you want your legacy to be?

This isn't a question that should be future-dated or something you should start thinking about when you retire. You should think about it and act upon your thoughts right now. Save us all from the awkward life crisis down the track and live purposefully now.

It's not rocket science that if you spend a huge portion of your life doing something that makes you feel good and brings you meaning, you're going to be a hell of a lot happier. Research shows that people who do work that they consider to be meaningful generally have higher levels of happiness and contentment in life.

If you feel a longing to do something else, start by looking at who is doing what you would love to do:

- Make a list of the people who are doing what you'd love to do.
- Do some research on how they got to where they are; what courses, qualifications or experience they built up to pursue that life and see if it's something that sounds up your alley.
- If possible, reach out to them and see if they'd be open to a coffee or an online meeting. (Think about what you could do for them in return, and don't be one of those people who asks, 'Can I pick your brain?' It's an awful phrase, lacking in generosity, and feels quite self-serving – as though this relationship will be a one-way street.)

Find your sharpest tool

What is it that you're really good at?

You don't have to completely change everything to do something that matters. There will often be an opportunity for you to do good and make positive change with the skills and attributes you already possess.

As my friend Sam McLean, the former head of GetUp, says, it's about using your sharpest tool to create change. Contributing in a way that is purposeful, helpful and aligned with your talents. You might be a great marketer or a great communicator; perhaps you're really good at logistics or coordinating a crowd; maybe you're a great artist or musician or a masterful educator. Look to your strengths and how you could use them to create change in your community or help the causes you are passionate about.

Other ways you can give that don't require you running off to live in the Amazon to fight against deforestation (although that would be pretty rad – if you do it, can we be friends?) might include:

- Looking at ways your workplace or business could drive real and meaningful change in the community.

- Joining a campaign you're passionate about and seeing how you could help with your skills.

- Going back to your school and giving a talk. See if there is a high-school student you could mentor.

- Connecting with your uni lecturers or teachers at your TAFE and offering to come back and do a tutorial or lecture with the students.

Warm sunshiny
people are
the best people.

Don't give away any of your precious energy to those who don't deserve it.

Surround yourself with people who feel like sunshine

There was a great line in the TV series *The Marvelous Mrs. Maisel*, when Midge Maisel's father says to her, 'You have to pick your friends as if there's a war going on.' That line has really stuck with me: who would you want to take into battle with you? Choose people who would have the strength and conviction to be there for you and with you in the very worst times.

And it's been one of the biggest learnings for me from the whole experience with cancer and recovery. Distance yourself from people who are not kind, who don't lift you up, love you, make your heart soar and bring out the absolute best in you. Life is too short to be around people who drain your energy and demand too much of your attention, and I can guarantee that when it all hits the fan the fairweather friends will not be there. If you don't feel you have wonderful people in your life yet, go find them. Volunteer, get involved with your community, join a sports team; they'll be out there, but sometimes it takes a bit of searching.

Life is too short to be around people who don't lift you up.

And a word about cool kids. Author Matt Haig tweeted:

Never be cool. Never try and be cool.
Never worry what the cool people think.
Head for the warm people. Life is warmth.
You'll be cool when you're dead.

Gosh, I love this. You know the people who are too cool to talk to you, smile, make you feel welcome; too cool to introduce themselves to you when you walk into a room or to remember your name after the sixth time they've met you. They're not cool, they're just bad mannered, often insecure or just plain arseholes (unless they have prosopagnosia – a condition where you cannot recognise faces – then they're excused). Here is the freeing part: you don't need them in your life. They add very little value.

It's funny how intimidating or unnerving these people can be; as though they hold some strange power, so you try harder to please them. These days post-cancer I just don't have the time for cool kids. I'm always kind, but if someone has bad energy or is an energy drain, they ain't taking any of my precious limited-edition energy. I don't care if they are rich, successful, well connected, drop-dead gorgeous. If they don't make me feel good they're not worth my energy – unless they're Brad Pitt, who, coincidentally, claims he has prosopagnosia.

So who are the most important people in your life? And do they get the very best of you?

Celebrate like crazy when you make another lap around the sun

There are two types of people in the world: those who love birthdays and those who hate them. Whether or not you like having a fuss made of you (we all have that friend who thinks their birthday lasts for a month of festivities) or would prefer no one to know about it, getting another lap around the sun is definitely something to cherish.

My very wise family friend Andrea totally changed my perception of ageing some years ago. Tragically Andrea and her husband Peter lost their divine daughter Jarrah in a bus accident while she was travelling through Africa. She was working there as a vet, helping local women look after their livestock better so they could be financially independent and support their families. Jarrah was a sunbeam of a human who was purpose-driven and focused on living a meaningful and intentional life, and her death was devastating to all who loved her, including her wonderful siblings. She was just 26 years old.

One night, many years before I was diagnosed, I was sitting beside Andrea at a birthday party. The person whose birthday it was, was lamenting turning another year older. Andrea turned to me and said,

'I think it's such a shame when people complain about their birthdays. A birthday is something to be celebrated. It means you got the gift of another year.'

It changed my approach to ageing and birthdays forever. So many people are denied the privilege of growing older.

When you get worried about getting older or start dreading another birthday; when you think, 'OMG is that a wrinkle?'; when you get caught up in all these silly, trivial, unimportant details that we think define us and that sometimes can consume us: remember, ageing is a luxury.

What really matters is that today you are here. Your heart beats, your lungs are breathing and you have the privilege of walking around in this magical and crazy world. Some days might be harder than others, but today you're here and you can do whatever you want with this day. Think about how lucky you are to have reached an age where wrinkles adorn your face. Sure, I still don't exactly want to roll out the red carpet to the wrinkles, but when I see one appear now I think, 'Hello fun lines! Gosh, we've sure had some good times.'

 NINJA TIP *If you don't like making a song and dance about your birthday or find it awkward having people celebrate with you, think about what would make this day memorable for you. Go for a hike; see some live music or a show; or treat yourself to a day of self-care. Do something that energises you to mark the celebration of the gift of another year.*

Enjoy this simple fleeting moment

We spend a lot of our time thinking about the future. Something that helps ground me when my thoughts are running away, is that in many years from now I'll give anything to be back here in this ordinary moment.

Perhaps you're not happy with the way your body looks, or where you're at right now, but in years to come, imagine how much you'd love to experience what you have right here and now. Imagine when you're 90, what you might give to have a day in your body just as it is right now. Maybe you're sitting around the living room with your family and you're feeling a bit annoyed or frustrated at someone, yet imagine if that someone you loved had passed on, what you might give to be back in this simple moment.

I made a pact with myself years ago to never get annoyed on the phone at my parents when they called. I hear so many people speak so poorly to their mums or dads when they call lovingly. I realised one day, when I was being a little short on the phone to my mum after a long day at work, that some day my beautiful mum won't be around to call me. The thought of that nearly broke my heart, so why wouldn't I just enjoy a conversation with her right now?

All we have is the moment we are in right now, that's it. So often we're grasping for the future and we miss the beauty in front of us. For me, it's been one of the biggest learnings to find more moments to be present and to enjoy what is right here, right now. (I'm definitely still a total rookie at this, but trying daily.)

This moment
is all we have.

Looking after our two homes

It's been a few years now since my life flipped upside down one very normal Thursday morning. People always ask, has it changed you?

My answer to that is ... *yes and no.*

It's changed me in many ways, but so many of those shifts have been about rediscovering what I already knew. Like finding lost rooms inside me that I forgot about long ago in the busyness of life. Cancer gave me a chance to reconnect and really listen to what I wanted.

To come home.

Priorities shift; you have a new-found appreciation for how short and fleeting and precious life is, and you question the way you want to spend the remainder of your time on Earth. Ultimately, for me, it's crystallised my desire to use my time purposefully.

To do something that matters with my life.

I've realised that the way we treat our bodies is reflected in the way we treat our planet. We live in a culture that is not in balance: it is all about taking, depleting, extracting. Getting maximum bang for our bucks, squeezing as much as we can out of our bodies, our time, our land, our waterways, our environment. We wait for a crisis before we act. A burnout, an illness, a horrific bushfire season, a species on the brink of collapse.

I was discussing this parallel recently with my good friend Anna Rose, a tireless climate campaigner. She said that we live in a culture that is extractive and not regenerative, and that if we are to progress as a society we need to get better at listening. Listening to our bodies and to the Earth. When there's a problem they usually tell us.

So many people ignore the signs that their bodies need them to stop and take care of them, just as we ignore the obvious signs the Earth is sending us that our one planet is in trouble.

Just like there's no Planet B, there's no Body B: we have to look after the one we've got.

Without a thriving and healthy environment, humans are completely stuffed. It's what our First Nations sisters and brothers have always known and practised: that harmony and balance are paramount. Recently, I was lucky enough to spend some time with Karrina Nolan, an Aboriginal woman who runs Original Power, an incredible organisation that works to build the power of Aboriginal and Torres Strait Islander peoples to protect Country. She shares the saying: 'If we have a sick Earth, we have sick people.'

We see ourselves as separate from nature, yet those trees that fill us with awe and wonder are our lungs. The Earth gives us all the sustenance we need to survive: water, food and oxygen. Not to mention joy and soul refreshment. But we humans don't quite get it. As the joke goes, 'If only trees gave out wi-fi, we'd probably plant so many we'd save the world.'

As I choked on bushfire smoke in Sydney in the summer of 2019–20, despite the fact the fires were raging many miles away, this was brought home in stark reality. Our country was ravaged by the worst fires in living history. An estimated three billion animals were killed. Over 12 million hectares burned: that's nearly the size of all of England's land area. An estimated 11.3 million Australians were affected by the smoke. I saw friends suffering with respiratory problems and mental health issues; families with young children locked inside for weeks. The most crucial thing we need to sustain us, clean air – the thing we take for granted every single day – was now no longer a given. The thick smoke was inescapable.

The warning light is flashing in our two homes: our bodies and our planet.

Yes, the obstacles can feel overwhelming, but as when someone gets a cancer diagnosis, we don't sit by and just give up and say, 'Oh well, that's too bad.' No, we do everything that we can to fight to preserve life: we act straight away and throw everything we've got at it.

A richer, more fulfilling and beautiful experience of life on Earth awaits us. One that is deeply nourishing, healing and regenerative for our lives and communities, as well as the animals and ecosystems we share our home with. We already have all the solutions we need to solve the climate crisis, to regenerate our lands and clean our oceans, and great progress is being made in every corner of the globe. We can move from a world of depletion and burnout to one of abundance and regeneration. That's an exciting future I want to be a part of (and it sounds a lot of fun).

Be bold with your life

I certainly don't have it all figured out, hell no, but I want to live this next chapter of my story boldly. I've realised that life is about enjoying the ride with people you love and doing something that matters with this fleeting time you have on Earth.

You don't have to wait for a giant shake-up to start really living a life you are proud of. You can start now.

We're all going to have surprise twists in life that will knock the wind out of us. While we would never choose them, often the hardest things that happen to us are strengthening us and shaping us in ways we can't even see or understand yet.

You already have everything you need inside you to deal with the challenges life will throw your way.

So be bold with this precious, glorious life you've been given.

ALL YOU GET IS THIS ONE LIFE

That is it. This is not a dress rehearsal.
This is the real deal.

So be bold with your life, surround
yourself with only the best.

Put your energy into the things
that really matter.

Treat the most important people
in your life as though they are the most
important people in your life.

Worry less about what others think.

Be kinder than you need to be
and grateful for all you have.

Love your body and appreciate
what it allows you to do.
Remember that ageing is a luxury.

Laugh more, have a damn
good time and remember that
there is always time for joy.

Leave the world better
than you found it.

Remember that it's never
too late to start.

And, above all else, look for the magic
all around you, right here, right now.

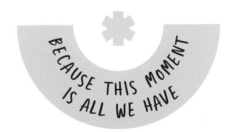

BECAUSE THIS MOMENT
IS ALL WE HAVE

Resources

MY FAVOURITE FEEL-GOOD THINGS

Watch, listen and read

For a list of my favourite laugh-out-loud TV shows, books, films and podcasts that will keep you giggling, go to **brionybenjamin.com.au**

Songs to make you feel inspired and good

For a kick-arse playlist to lift your spirits, you'll find my 'Life Is Tough, But So Are You' playlist at **brionybenjamin.com.au**

TED Talks to keep you inspired

- *We don't 'move on' from grief. We move forward with it.* Nora McInerny (TEDWomen 2018)

- *Before I die I want to ...* Candy Chang (TEDGlobal 2012)

- *The power of vulnerability.* Brené Brown (TEDXHouston, June 2010)

- *Your body language may shape who you are.* Amy Cuddy (TEDGlobal 2012)

- *Do schools kill creativity?* Sir Ken Robinson (TED2006)

Beautiful poems to calm the mind

- 'Desiderata' Max Ehrmann (1927)

- 'The Peace of Wild Things' Wendell Berry, *New Collected Poems* (Counterpoint, 2012)

- 'What is Success' Bessy A. Stanley, *More Heart Throbs Volume 2* (Chapple Publishing Company, 1911)

Great gift ideas

For links to some amazing gift ideas for anyone going through a tough time, go to **brionybenjamin.com.au**

EMERGENCY HELPLINES

Lifeline 13 11 14; lifeline.org.au
24-hour crisis support and suicide-prevention services. They exist so that no Australian has to experience their darkest time alone. Give them a buzz if you would like to chat to someone.

Beyond Blue 1300 22 46 36; beyondblue.org.au
Beyond Blue has trained mental health professionals you can chat to 24 hours a day, 7 days a week. It's a great starting point if you'd like some guidance about what to do next.

Suicide Call Back Service 1300 659 467; suicidecallbackservice.org.au
If you or someone you know is feeling overwhelmed and suicidal call the helpline, or chat via text or video on their website. You can speak with a qualified professional counsellor, social worker or psychologist, trained to listen, understand you, and help you find ways to feel better.

Cancer Council 13 11 20; cancer.org.au
A free and confidential telephone support service for people experiencing cancer and those who are supporting them. (A friend used this service and it made a huge difference to how they supported me.)

1800 RESPECT 1800 737 732; 1800respect.org.au
If you or someone you know is at risk or in an abusive relationship, you can call at any time or chat online.

Kids Helpline 1800 55 1800; kidshelpline.com.au
Phone and online counselling services for kids, teens, young adults, parents and teachers.

Legal services
For a list of free legal services in Australia check out the resources at **probonocentre.org.au/legal-help/legal-aid/**

Lifeline 0800 543 354 (0800 LIFELINE); lifeline.org.nz

Women's refuge 0800 733 843 (0800 REFUGE); womensrefuge.org.nz

Good Samaritans 116 123; samaritans.org

Supportline 01708 765 200; supportline.org.uk

National Domestic Abuse Helpline
0808 2000 247; nationaldahelpline.org.uk

The Lifeline national suicide prevention line 1800 273 8255 (1800 273 TALK); suicidepreventionlifeline.org

Crisis Text Line Text HOME to 741 741; crisistextline.org

National Domestic Violence Hotline 1800 799 7233 (1800 799 SAFE) or TTY 1800 787 3224; thehotline.org

Lymphoma

Lymphoma is a common cancer. Symptoms can include night sweats, weight loss, swollen lymph nodes, itchy skin and exhaustion. For more information on lymphoma and other cancers go to:
cancer.org.au
leukaemia.org.au
lymphoma.org.au

REFERENCES

Section 1

page 16 Kaplan, Justin, ed., 'Reinhold Niebuhr (1892–1971)', *Bartlett's Familiar Quotations* (Hachette, 17th ed., 2002) p 735.

page 20 Tedeschi, Richard G. and Calhoun, Lawrence G., 'Posttraumatic Growth: Conceptual Foundations and Empirical Evidence', *Psychological Inquiry*, January 2004, Vol. 15, no. 1, pp 1-18.

Section 2

page 45 Seligman, Martin E.P., *Learned Optimism: How to Change Your Mind and Your Life* (Pocket Books, 1991).

Section 3

page 54 headspace.com

page 56 Dooley, Roger, 'Why Faking a Smile Is a Good Thing', *Forbes*, 26 February 2013; van Cuylenberg, Hugh, *The Resilience Project: Finding Happiness through Gratitude, Empathy and Mindfulness* (Random House Australia, 2019)

page 58 Cameron, Julia, and Bryan, Mark, *The Artist's Way: A Spiritual Path to Higher Creativity* (Perigee, 1992); Phelan, Hayley, 'What's all this about journalling?', *The New York Times*, 25 October 2018; Rodriguez, Tori, 'Writing can help injuries heal faster', *Scientific American*, 1 November 2013.

page 62 Mills, Paul J. et al., 'The Role of Gratitude in Well-being in Asymptomatic Heart Failure Patients', *Integrative Medicine: A Clinician's Journal*, 2015, Vol. 14, no. 1, p 51; Allen, Summer, 'The Science of Gratitude', white paper, Greater Good Science Center UC Berkeley, May 2018.

page 63 Konish, Lorie, 'This is the real reason most Americans file for bankruptcy', *CNBC* 'Personal Finance', 11 February 2019.

page 68 Haas, Susan Biali, 'Working with your hands does wonders for your brain', *Psychology Today*, 21 June 2019.

Section 5

page 88 Emerson, Ralph Waldo, 'Education' *The Complete Writings of RWE* Vol 2, ed. Edward Emerson (W.H. Wise & Co, 1929).

Section 6

page 113 motherteresa.org

page 114 Ulrich, R.S., 'View through a window may influence recovery from surgery', *Science, New Series*, 1984, Vol. 224, no. 4647, pp 420–21; Williams, F., *The Nature Fix: Why nature makes us happier, healthier, and more creative* (W.W. Norton, 2017).

page 115 Nagasawa, Miho, et al., 'Dog's gaze at its owner increases owner's urinary oxytocin during social interaction', *Hormones and Behavior*, 2009, Vol. 55, no. 3, pp 434–41.

Section 7

page 120 Silk, Susan and Goldman, Barry, 'How not to say the wrong thing', *Los Angeles Times*, 7 April 2013.

page 129 McDowell, Emily, excerpt from God's Plan Empathy Card. Available at emandfriends.com © Knock Knock LLC

Section 8

page 152 Jackson, Gabrielle, *Pain and Prejudice: A call to arms for women and their bodies* (Allen & Unwin, 2019); Nabel, Elizabeth G., M.D., 'Coronary heart disease in women – An ounce of prevention', *New England Journal of Medicine*, 24 August 2000, Vol. 343, no. 8, pp 572–74.

page 156 cancer.org.au/cancer-information/causes-and-prevention/ diet-and-exercise/move-your-body.

page 157 Rucklidge, Julia, 'The surprisingly dramatic role of nutrition in mental health', TEDxChristchurch 2014; cancer.org.au/cancer-information/ causes-and-prevention/diet-and-exercise/meat-and-cancer-risk; 'IARC monographs evaluate consumption of red meat and processed meat', International Agency for Research on Cancer press release No. 240, 26 October 2015.

page 158 Walker, Matthew, *Why We Sleep: Unlocking the Power of Sleep and Dreams* (Scribner, 2017).

pages 158–159 'Research shows bad relationships can also mean bad health', *Forbes* 'Quora', 3 May, 2018.

page 159 de Sales, St Francis, *The Spiritual Letters of St Francis de Sales* (Rivingtons, 1871).

page 164 Walker, Matthew, *Why We Sleep: Unlocking the Power of Sleep and Dreams* (Scribner, 2017).

Section 9

page 178 Rosso, Brent D., Dekas, Kathryn H., and Wrzesniewski, Amy, 'On the meaning of work: A theoretical integration and review', *Research in Organizational Behavior*, 2010, Vol. 30, pp 91–127.

page 183 Haig, Matt, *Reasons to Stay Alive* (Canongate Books, 2015)

Thanks to these legends

To my brilliant publisher Kelly Doust, thank you for this extraordinary opportunity. I loved you from the minute I met you. Thank you for being such a radiant, divine, supportive woman; for making the process joyful and fun; and for giving me the confidence that I could write this book. The whole team at Murdoch Books – what a glorious bunch: Lou for believing in the idea from the start, Virginia my wonderful editor, Melody for making my words sing, Trisha and Susanne for your lovely design, Kristy for overseeing the beautiful design work and to Sue the PR queen. Thank you for bringing my book into the world.

To my amazing family, the best support crew a girl could ask for. Denise: my brilliant mother, superwoman and bliss-ball queen. Thank you for holding my hand every single step of the way through cancer and this book! My wonderful dad, Anthony, for all your support, love and vet advice. To my darling sisters, the twinnies: Molly, who jumped straight on a plane from London to be with me, and Rhi, who was the first to crack an excellent inappropriate joke. Thanks for all of the laughs, love and sage advice. And Enzo you little darling of a dog, I'll love you forever.

To my extraordinary doctors, nurses and the medical admin staff who supported me through treatment. Especially Annmarie Bosco, Tara Cochrane, Bill Ledger and my legendary nurses Amy, Jodi and many more.

My best friend Nikki for being the most sunshine you could ever meet in a human. To Clare Bear, for creating a beautiful film out of the mess of footage I gave you, which led to this book, and for all your creative guidance. To Jenna, thank you for your beautiful book of thoughts you sent me, which helped me so much in my journey. To Bill Manos, for your belief and support always. To Natasha, Tim, David, Rohan, Jess, Danny and Victoria, I treasure our friendship. And to all my beautiful ASAS girls for your support. To Marieke, for inspiring this whole journey by sending me *The Artist's Way* and reminding me of my love of writing. To Roger, head of crisis logistics and planning for rallying all the troops during my treatment. To Henry Carroll for your writing guidance (and for being the first to congratulate me on getting cancer – LOL).

To Mia Freedman for being a champion of women; for giving me an amazing opportunity at Mamamia; for trusting me wholeheartedly; and for being fierce in your fight for women and the causes you so passionately support. And to my entire Mamamia family, thanks for all the sparkle, love (and blood donations).

Thank you Sandy Peacock, Clare Stephens, Holly Wainwright and Leigh Campbell for all your encouragement on my early drafts, and Amanda Lo Teer for all your guidance and support through the creative process.

To all my beautiful SPL Squash buddies for your support, community and encouragement always.

To my new friends I met through Lymphoma: Emily, Rikki, Maddie, Nat, Steph, Krystal, Steph and Nicole. You are beautiful warrior women doing great things in the world.

Thanks to all my wonderful teachers over the years: for inspiring a love of literature and writing, especially Naomi Middlebrook and Sheree Dwyer.

To all the people who have followed my story; who sent messages of love and support; and who shared your stories with me and encouraged me to keep sharing mine, thank you.

And finally a huge thanks to you, the dear reader holding this book right now. Thanks for giving me the gift of having my words and thoughts read. In many ways this book has helped bring me back to myself, to make sense of it all and kick off the next chapter of my life. So thank you for buying something I have created from my heart. I really hope it has helped you with whatever journey you are on.

I wish you all the love and strength. Remember: you've got this. Xx

Published in 2021 by Murdoch Books, an imprint of Allen & Unwin

Murdoch Books Australia
83 Alexander Street
Crows Nest NSW 2065
Phone: +61 (0)2 8425 0100
murdochbooks.com.au
info@murdochbooks.com.au

Murdoch Books UK
Ormond House
26–27 Boswell Street
London WC1N 3JZ
Phone: +44 (0) 20 8785 5995
murdochbooks.co.uk
info@murdochbooks.co.uk

For corporate orders and custom publishing, contact our business development team at
salesenquiries@murdochbooks.com.au

Publisher: Kelly Doust
Editorial Manager: Virginia Birch
Design Manager: Kristy Allen
Designer: Trisha Garner and Susanne Geppert
Cover Designer: Trisha Garner
Editor: Melody Lord
Production Director: Lou Playfair

ISBN 978 1 92235 136 4 Australia
ISBN 978 1 91166 827 5 UK

A catalogue record for this
book is available from the
NATIONAL
LIBRARY
OF AUSTRALIA
National Library of Australia

A catalogue record for this book is available from the British Library

Colour reproduction by Splitting Image Colour Studio Pty Ltd, Clayton, Victoria
Printed by C&C Offset Printing Co. Ltd., China

10 9 8 7 6 5 4 3 2 1

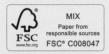